The Sun Always Rises

To Joann,
Thank-you
for Everything!
Love you!
Kelly
1-31-18

I believe we all need validation in our life no matter how strong or confident we are. And we should all have our "go to" people. Our go to people can be different people at different times in our life. And quite often they get as much from giving to us as we receive from them. As I have said before, I believe everyone is in our life for a reason, even if it's only for a season. I am very thankful and grateful for mine.

A special thank you to those who have shared their stories with me and have allowed me to share them with my readers, and to those who have inspired me and encouraged me to "feed my soul" by writing this book.

The Sun Always Rises
How to Thrive in Times of Loss

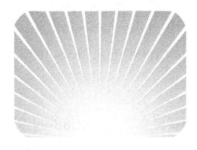

Kelly Lowe

CHB Media
Publisher

ISBN 978-1-946088-94-9

Front and Back Cover Photos by Kelly Lowe

CHB MEDIA, PUBLISHER

(386) 690-9295
chbmedia@gmail.com

CONTENTS

INTRODUCTION

I AM SO PLEASED THAT KELLY LOWE has decided to share her story of how she escaped the shadow of loss to discover a beautiful *new normal*. Her narrative is honest in its lows and optimistic in its highs, and is both personal and universal. Parts of it are unique to her, but most of what she describes will be familiar to all who have suffered a similar fate. Her revelations are simple—as life is often more simple than we make it—yet complex enough that she finds no need to gloss over very real challenges. I believe you'll find her guidance to be wise and easy to follow.

If you have suffered because a loved one who was there one moment is now suddenly gone, *The Sun Always Rises* will illuminate a path that can help you *thrive in a time of loss*. In such times thinking clearly can be difficult, and things that are pretty straight forward—even inevitable—may feel mind boggling or beyond solution. A counselor like Kelly who has suffered the same kinds of loss, understands human nature, and can articulate a clear vision of the way forward can be invaluable in stormy times. Kelly Lowe has a zest for life that shines through on every page. Beyond that, she knows the terrain of loss and recovery and speaks a language which talks directly to the wounded heart seeking to heal.

— Gary Broughman
Publisher, CHB Media

About Kelly Lowe

KELLY LOWE IS AN ASTROLOGICAL COUNSELOR, teacher, and author. She has been a professional astrological counselor for more than 30 years, helping her clients to better understand themselves, and to cope with challenging cycles in their lives.

Kelly believes that her faith in God and understanding of astrology have been the keys to recovering from her own losses and challenging cycles, including an early divorce, and the death of two wonderful husbands. Her life and journey are a testament to recovery and prosperity. Her joy is helping others do the same.

Kelly has appeared on national TV, been a regular guest on several radio shows, and publishes a monthly astrology newsletter. She has taught astrology at Seminole State College and Daytona State College, and gives frequent astrological lectures throughout the country. Her first book, *An Astrologer's Journey*, was recommended in reviews by leading national publications. Her monthly newsletter is available on her website at www.astrologytalk. com, and you can also visit her on Facebook.com/ astrologytalk.com.

"And as she fell apart, her shattered pieces began to bloom — blossoming until she became herself exactly as she was meant to be . . ." — Becca Lee (author)

Chapter One

A HEALING JOURNEY

Just about the time you think life is running great and you have everything under control, everything changes. The lesson, it seems, is that we should always expect to face the unexpected—for better or for worse. Apparently, having everything "under control" is just an illusion.

After three surgeries, one round of chemotherapy and radiation, my husband Tony and I lost the battle. His cancer metastasized. We fought it as hard and as long as we possibly could, with the help of all the medical experts and prayers that we could solicit, but the diagnosis was not a good one to begin with. Small bowel cancer is so rare that there has not been enough research done on it to have developed an effective treatment.

I learned that cancers that are more mainstream, such as breast cancer and colon cancer tend to get more funding for research and treatment development. I suppose this makes sense, but logic is seldom of any comfort when we find ourselves being swept downstream through life's rapids.

The doctors gave him the same chemo cocktail that they give colon cancer patients, which we were told was the best they had to offer. It was certainly not a sure thing by a long shot, but it never is—even when it's one of the more common cancers. Even after going through the side effects of chemo, there was no guarantee, but our oncologist told us that if it was his father, he would recommend going through this chemo protocol. That was all we needed to hear. It was good enough for us. But really, what choice did we have? There are times in life when, as hard as it might be, we are forced to give up our natural desire to be in control, and hand it over to the doctors, or maybe to God. This can be a very hard lesson to learn.

> I learned by doing it that writing was nurturing to my soul.

Even with the limited knowledge of this strain of cancer, believe me when I say we did everything we could to fight it. The survival rate after five years is only five percent. Of course we believed with all of our heart that we were going to be in that five percent.

It was during this time that I began my first book, *An Astrologer's Journey.* In January of 2011 Tony had just been diagnosed with cancer. Surgery was scheduled within days of the diagnosis because it is such an aggressive cancer. Surgery was followed by chemotherapy, beginning six weeks later. I choose to take the time while he was recovering and undergoing treatment to immerse myself in writing my book. It had been my dream and goal for many years, and I finally found the discipline to do it. I was feeling it, but it was also written in the stars.

I knew that Saturn, the planet that is the disciplinarian, the tester and the teacher was making his journey though my 3rd house, indicating a cycle of mental structure and discipline. When Saturn is traveling through this area of a person's chart it is important to be mentally structured and focused. And what better way to harness that energy then to tackle writing my first book.

I knew that my outside activities would be limited because I would be staying close to home during his treatment, so I felt it would be good therapy for me and for him. Writing kept me upbeat and in a positive frame of mind. I learned by doing it that writing was nurturing to my soul. Saturn, the teacher was serving me well. He was keeping me focused and working at home with a positive attitude as we were going through treatment for this rare and horrible disease.

I have always kept a journal since I was a little girl, but never did I write with the intention of anyone reading it. In fact, I plan to burn all of my journals before I die—if I get the chance anyway. I'm not sure exactly what day that will be, but here's hoping it will be many years in the future!

The writing of my first published book was different from writing my journals. It was written with the intent of sharing a story and information that I hoped would be motivational and helpful—and it was, for many people.

But I've written this book to "feed MY soul." If it also feeds your soul, that's a blessing.

My background is certainly very eclectic and diverse which is probably why I was motivated to share my struggles and adventures. But when my husband first passed away in June of 2015, I wasn't ready to openly write or even talk about it. I'm sure others who have suffered loss have experienced something similar. I wanted to, but I just couldn't bring myself to sit down at my computer and open my heart. It was too painful.

I remember reading a book a friend loaned to me soon after Tony's death called *Magical Thinking* by Joan Didion. Her husband had a fatal heart attack at the dinner table. Although she was already a renowned author, she wrote in her book that she was unable to write again for two years after her husband died. At the time I thought that was odd. Why two years? My husband had just passed away and I was still in a fog, but I didn't know it.

I thought I was doing just fine. He had been declining for a couple of years and I thought I was ready to heal and go on. Again, just as the cancer and its treatment had been beyond my control, so was the timing of my recovery. *I learned that it takes as long as it takes to heal . . . to find yourself again, or to reinvent yourself.*

TRANSITING JUPITER IN THE 3RD HOUSE

Then a little over a year after Tony passed, I was, of course, following my astrology chart and saw that Jupiter, the guardian angel and benefic, was about to begin her one-year journey through my third house of communication. I knew that if I was ever going to write another book, this would be the time. It was now or never. It was the right time to begin writing and sharing my healing journey—my journey of reinventing and rediscovering myself. And once I had begun the writing became a big part of the healing process.

To me, writing a book is like the old adage about eating an elephant—the only way to do it is one bite at a time. And once you start, the ideas and energy flow. It all comes together. I'd wake up at 4:30 in the morning with ideas and a need to write about the thoughts that are running through my head. So I've learned to keep a note pad next to my bed, and since I sleep alone I can turn the light on and write them down. Then eventually, I just started getting up at 5 a.m. and going to my computer.

Jupiter Retrograde Extends Opportunity

Fortunately, I knew that Jupiter was going to be going retrograde while it was traveling through my 3rd house of communications, which would extent her beneficial influence on my motivation to write. I knew I needed to take advantage of this cycle, and I could see by what was flowing out of me that the time had come to "get it down on paper." My healing journey had begun, but it wasn't an easy journey and for the first time in my life I truly understood the old saying, "two steps forward, one step back."

Life is never the same after losing a spouse, even when you are prepared and think that you are ready. Four years and seven months after my husband was diagnosed with small bowel cancer, after three surgeries and one round of chemo and a round of radiation treatment, it finally took over his body.

I guess I can be grateful for the three good years we had before the cancer metastasized. I'm certainly grateful for the fifteen wonderful years we shared together before his diagnosis. But it was difficult to keep sight of that as the pet scans where showing the fatal diagnosis.

Although I had already lost one husband to heart disease, it did not make losing Tony any easier. As I look back, I do feel blessed to have had two very special, wonderful men in my life, knowing many women never find one.

Both of my deceased husbands were very special men. They will be in my heart forever. I can close my eyes and see them, healthy and happy, sharing a laugh or lifting a glass of wine with me. And I remember the role each of them played in making me the woman I am today.

Although they were both Sagittarians, they were very different in their personalities. Larry had an 11th house sun, which tends to be a more social and outgoing personality. He loved a good party, enjoyed his friends, was a very active member of Rotary and enjoyed his MG car club friends. He was always ready to entertain.

Tony had a 12th house sun, which was an indication to me as an astrologer that he enjoyed his alone time, his solitude. Although he was charming and interactive in his profession, all he really wanted or needed was to be with me after he retired. I guess that is why it was so different after he passed. We pretty much did everything together, especially during his last few years with me. We traveled; we watched golf, tennis, football, and the Olympics on TV, and often went out to lunch or dinner. We enjoyed our time together. It was easy. It was comfortable. It was a great life until that nasty cancer reared its ugly head in his body.

At first it seemed so unfair. Why him? He had never really been sick a day from the time when I met him. He had good genes. Tony's father was in his late eighties when we first met. Tony was very active and healthy. He jogged, played golf, and worked out on his Boflex. This was very important to me, since my previous husband passed away at fifty-eight and his father also passed away at fifty-eight with a heart attack.

His mother had passed away with breast cancer when she was in her 50s, but we were told that breast cancer and small bowel are totally unrelated. Her cancer had not predisposed him to this. Of course, we never in our wildest imagination ever dreamed that he would get the Big "C" of any variety. Does anyone ever think about getting cancer? I know we didn't. I guess if you have a genetic predisposition that's one thing, and somehow easier to accept? Probably not. But who ever heard of getting small bowel cancer—whoever even heard of it at all?

This year, an estimated 10,190 adults (5,380 men and 4,810 women) in the United States will be diagnosed with small bowel cancer. It is estimated that 1,390 deaths (770 men and 620 women) from this disease will occur this year.

For comparison, colorectal cancer, the third most common cancer in both men and women in the United States, will be diagnosed 13 times as often. This year, an estimated 135,430 adults in the United States will be diagnosed with colorectal cancer. (*statistics, cancer.net*)

So, we were both shocked when he was diagnosed. As I noted earlier, our oncologist told us that there was no proven protocol treatment for it, since it was so rare. But they had been using a similar chemo formula that was used for colon cancer patients. The survival statistics were against us, even with chemo, and we knew the chemo was going to make him so sick. We were hesitant. But our oncologist told us that if it were him or his family member, he would encourage having the chemo.

The first step was surgery, and after a nasty, major surgery to remove the growing tumors, the surgeon declared he got it all. This was followed by a precautionary six months of chemo. Our lives changed dramatically during this time. He slowed down, lost a lot of weight, and I chose this time to begin my first book while taking care of him.

I LOST MY JOB

When he passed there was such a huge void in my life. I felt like I had lost my job. My job for the previous five years—the five years since his cancer was first diagnosed—was to take care of him. We had three good years in that time before the cancer came roaring back, and for that I'm thankful. But even then I was focused on Tony.

CHANGES IN LATITUDE, CHANGES IN ATTITUDE

Travel is always a good distraction or antidote to help in the healing process—or at least I thought it would be. My first trip was to San Diego to visit my aunt and uncle about six months after Tony passed away. I did the very same thing when Larry passed away.

Traveling, getting away, escaping—"changes in

latitude, changes in attitude," as the Jimmy Buffett song goes—was my first instinct. But unfortunately, no matter where you go, there you are. I couldn't run away from the feeling of loss deep in the pit of my stomach. The memories and heartbreak followed me no matter where I was.

He was always in my DNA, always in the back of my mind and my memory bank. There was that feeling of being disconnected. I remember on my first trip after he passed, I really missed calling him first thing in the morning as I had when I woke up on previous trips to California before his death. I'd wake up at 5 or 6 a.m. when it was 8 or 9 a.m. in Florida. I'd usually catch him as he was on his way to the golf course.

I'll never forget the day I found out "it" was back.

Tony did enjoy his time to himself and didn't mind if I was away on a speaking engagement or visiting family. But he was always happy to hear my voice when I called, just as I was happy to hear his.

Tony was born with his sun in the 12th house. People who have their sun in the 12th house in their astrological chart tend to enjoy their solitary time. I think that was one of the reasons we got along so well right from the very beginning. I gave him the space and time that he needed for himself. And my 9th house sun loved and needed space and freedom and independence. I loved to travel and so did he, so we had a good balance of time together and apart.

We certainly did our share of traveling before his diagnosis. But after that we were always afraid to plan anything too far in advance. We never knew when that PET scan was going to bring us bad news, as it eventually did.

I'll never forget the day I found out "it" was back. He had gone in for one of his routine follow-up appointments with his oncologist while I was away. My son had taken my grandson and me on a cruise for my birthday. Tony was not a cruiser. Even ferry boats made him seasick. This cruise was just a long weekend to Mexico—a bonding time for my son, grandson and me. It was a beautiful opportunity and I was smiling inside.

I did try to get Tony to reschedule his oncology appointment until after my return. I had been to every single one of his oncologist appointments with him. They were always fine when I was there. No change until this one, like it had somehow snuck through in my absence.

I was driving home from the cruise when I called home and he gave me the bad news. He said the PET scan showed spots. I felt like someone had hit me in the stomach and knocked all the wind out of my lungs.

At that time we didn't even know the extent of what "spots" really meant, or just how bad it was. It was when I went with him to his next appointment that we learned that the cancer had metastasized. There were several spots—as the doctor called them—and when he mentioned the liver and lungs I knew it was not good. Little did we know that that Tony would be gone in less than two years.

Fortunately we did enjoy our life—the many things we did together including traveling—prior to cancer hitting us. I say *us* because it was a major life change for both of us.

Everyone loses or has lost someone at one time or another in their life. It would be impossible to go through this life without experiencing that pain—the pain of the loss of a loved one or a friend. Some of us have felt that pain many more times than others. It seems that no matter how many times we experience it, the hurt and healing is something that we have to go through. Unfortunately it is a very personal process. No one can do it for us. No one can carry the cross. No one can cry our tears. No one can stop the heartaches. No one can convince you that the sun always rises until at long last you see it inching above the horizon. And no one can make the pain go away any faster than the healing of time will allow. Healing is a journey. It is a sad, lonely journey that we each process and deal with in our own private special way.

Everyone deals with loss in their own way and in their own time ... and among the many things that makes each of us different, I have learned that each sun sign has their own way of dealing with their loss, which I will talk about later.

In true Aries fashion, within a week of his passing I had all of the furniture removed from his office, which is where the hospital bed had been. I had the room painted and went out and bought a very comfortable queen size bed. I have turned his office into an official guest room which is something we never had before—his office had a sofa bed which doubled as a guest room. My grandson is thoroughly enjoying the new bed. And I so enjoy his visits.

FROM PURPOSE TO NEW PURPOSE

I believe that the magnitude and duration of the

healing process depends a great deal on the role we had in the daily life of the person who passed on. For example, in my case I was my husband's caregiver for the months leading up to his passing. He filled the major part of my life and my daily routine. He was my foremost purpose and in the forefront on my mind at all times.

When he finally lost his battle with small bowel cancer I felt I had lost my purpose in life. My purpose was to take care of him—take him to his doctor's appointments, prepare his meals, keep him company. We watched all the golf tournaments and tennis matches together. He especially loved the major golf tournaments. Before his cancer started getting the best of him, he enjoyed playing golf a couple times each week. In fact, he was the reason I learned to play. It wasn't too long after we started dating that I decided that it would probably be a good idea if I learned to play. And as it turned out, it was a great idea.

We enjoyed many wonderful golfing vacations together. He especially loved playing the courses in Scottsdale, Arizona. Although the summers are brutally hot, we would stay on our Eastern Time Zone schedule and get up 4 a.m. for a 6 a.m. tee time. We watched many sunrises over the desert.

Memories . . . they are wonderful and I'm told they are part of the healing process. Yes, it is a process. Wouldn't it be wonderful if you could just open a can of "heal yourself" and all of the pain and sorrow would be gone, sort of a "pain no more" remedy?

But we all know that just isn't the way it works. It's a slow journey, and I the amount of time that it takes depends not only on your closeness in the last days, weeks, months or years, but also on the depth of your relationship before the illness. I know that my husband's adult daughters, who live out of town, spoke with him every day on the phone. So he was a daily part of their life, even if just for thirty minutes. His sister talked with him every day over the phone about the stock market. She said that when he left she lost her enthusiasm and interest in the market. It just wasn't the without him.

It's said that the loss of a spouse or child is one of the most difficult things that you can go through. I tend to agree with that to a certain point, but having also lost both of my parents I can still recall the pain and deep sense of loss. I guess we expect that our parents are going to die before us, but we don't think of our spouse or children ever dying—unless of course they are diagnosed with cancer. Then we live with that fear looming over our head every day. We dig deep into our emotional reservoir and learn the meaning of the saying, "Make the most of every day."

As I approached the one year mark after his passing, those life memories of *us* began to find their way back into my consciousness. Most of them were beautiful, but the sad final days were there as well. In either case it seemed as if Tony was there, again holding my hand, giving me faith and courage to take the next step, and to enjoy each new sunrise. Watching the sun rise over the Atlantic in those early dark days built my confidence, and continues to do so today.

"You won't die in the middle of the night if you've got something in the morning that you've got to do." — Carl Ryner

Chapter Two

FINDING THE NEW NORMAL

In my first book I discussed the path I followed to astrology. It was a path with many stops along the way, including meditation and traditional religion. Always, the search was for a way to get in touch with myself and understand why I felt the way I did, and how I fit into the order of the universe. Astrology gave me a way of *seeing* that made the most sense to me. First off, I learned that by following the lunar cycle I could better understand and appreciate my emotions and the cycles of my emotions.

When my love and interest in astrology began back in the early 1980s, I was single and looking for my prince charming. This was during the era when Linda Goodman's sun sign book had just come out and Nancy Reagan's use of astrology became public knowledge. Yes, for those of you who don't remember or were not yet born, it was quite a big deal when it first was revealed that Nancy Reagan was consulting with an astrologer to help President Ronald Reagan.

Timing is everything and astrology can be a valuable tool to help select the best time to achieve the best results, so I assumed she consulted her astrologer to help him with timing for scheduling his various meetings so that he would get the best possible results.

I was delighted when I had the opportunity to attend one of Linda Goodman's astrology talks at a major conference back in the 80s when I was a student of astrology—not that we ever stop learning, but I was a novice back then.

My personal interest and studies began as a hobby and developed into a career. Along the way, I was blessed and fortunate that I did meet two "prince charmings." Although I lost both of them, after I was left alone I felt very fortunate that I had an interest and a career that I was passionate about.

When Tony and I first moved to the beach in 2012, after he retired, I sort of put my career on the back burner. I cut back on my consultation appointments and did not really connect professionally with our new community. I was more involved and focused on decorating our new home, entertaining our families, and traveling.

Life was good. He was my prince and I was his princess. We enjoyed our new home and our new retired life. And he, at that time, was in perfect health. He exercised regularly, ate a healthy diet, never smoked and only drank wine occasionally. He had a great attitude about life. He always saw the glass half full rather than half empty. He was the epitome of a Sagittarian. He was my soul mate and we led a charmed life together.

So when he was diagnosed in November of 2010 with the cancer that would later take his life, you could have knocked me over with a feather. I was devastated to say the least. I have already spoken of how this changed my life and his, keeping us closer to home than we had become accustomed to as the happy travelers.

So with this new challenge came an opportunity—a chance to write the book I'd been thinking about for so long. This time while I was taking care of him would be my time to write, and to feed my soul. Writing became my window to the world, my haven, my motivation. Life was still good because he was still there with me. He had a great attitude and spirit even when he was recovering from his surgery and going through chemo. And I was happy to be there, writing *An Astrologer's Journey, My Life With the Stars* and taking care of my husband.

My book was published in November of 2011, one year after his diagnosis. I was so happy that he was able to come to my first book signing. We continued to live a relatively normal life after he completed his treatment. By that time frequent and regular follow-up tests and visits with his oncologist had come to feel normal. Then, three years into his remission, the devastating blow struck us. His cancer had metastasized. There were spots on his liver, small bowel, and lung. This was not good.

Another surgery was scheduled, followed by radiation for the spot on his lung. Unfortunately, this was the beginning of the end for us. I was once again going to lose my prince charming.

After a long and tedious journey, I was reeling with emotions and trying to find my new normal. Yes, there is still a period of shock and disbelief even when you know the end is inevitable. Even though I knew it was coming and could see the handwriting on the wall, it still didn't make it any easier. So when he was gone I did the only thing I knew how to do—I threw myself back into my work and "came out of the closet" in my local community.

I started scheduling local workshops and talks. I joined the local Chamber of Commerce. I not only joined, but I became very active and involved. I joined a networking leads group that met once a week. And I went to all the ribbon cuttings and after hours social events. Now granted, this would not be a healing therapy for everyone, but it seemed to work for me.

> For me, going through the healing and grieving process needed to be accelerated.

Maybe it was the answer to my prayers. I can remember sitting out by the pool one day at my son's house, not too long after Tony passed away, watching the sunrise shimmering through the trees. It made me think of God and feel his presence. I started speaking to God.

"Help me find to my path and direction as I travel through this new journey. Help me to be clear minded and to be a better person and know that You are always with me. I am never alone. I feel Your presence as I am looking through the trees at the sunrise."

I actually wrote this in my journey that morning which is why I remembered it so clearly. Yes, I kept a journal which is one of the things that is strongly recommended when dealing with a loss. It's a wonderful way to process your feelings and move through the healing journey.

INTRODUCTION TO BAUD THERAPY

It wasn't long after my conversation with God that the psychologist I was seeing for grief counseling introduced me to a treatment called BAUD, which is a Bio Acoustical Utilization Device. This is a relatively new neurological treatment that is used for "reset therapy." My therapist's father, Dr. George Lindenfeld, was instrumental in researching and developing this technique.

This treatment is very cutting edge and involves sound waves and using a headset. I must admit that I was a little leery of being a part of something that was so newly developed without much of track record in the field. But at the same time it was also an exciting idea to be part of a new therapy. And since I am an adventurous, pioneering Aries, I thought *why not*? I was suffering from so much pain and depression that I was willing to try anything that might help speed up the healing process. Besides, Aries are always eager to do things fast. For me, going through the healing and grieving process needed to be accelerated.

Fast doesn't always mean easy. It was very emotionally draining and painful in the beginning, but I could see that progress was being made as the treatments continued. In the beginning I cried even more that I had in the days and weeks after his death. But there in-between the tears was a feeling of peace and serenity. I stayed with this treatment for several weeks, and when that time was up I knew I had made progress on my journey. Yes it was fast, which was exactly what I was looking for and needed.

Dr. Lindenfeld is very passionate about getting the information about this treatment out to the public but only under the right circumstances. My therapist feels strongly that BAUD therapy should only be approached under the supervision and guidance of a professional who is trained and certified in the technique. For more information, you can check out this website. BAUD is a Powerful Therapy Tool. http://baudtherapy.com/studies.html

The treatment helped me through the recovery period when I couldn't stop crying. I'd wake up crying and I'd fall asleep crying. I was fortunate to find an excellent psychologist in my hometown who was trained in this treatment, considering that there are only 210 trained BAUD therapists in the entire country.

I believe the treatment saved me months of extended crying and depression. Not that grieving and depression aren't normal or necessary after experiencing a loss, I just found this treatment to be a great aid and tool to help me to process my emotions. It was a tremendous release mechanism. As painful as it was in the beginning, it was well worth the time and energy it took.

I don't know how I would have felt had I not gone through the treatment or what my time frame would have been to return to a "normal" life without crying every day, but I believe it was an invaluable tool to help me through the healing journey. Maybe I would have discovered another therapy that would

Kelly Lowe

have helped, but I do know this: recovery is only possible if you participate in the process. That might require taking chances, taking a leap of faith and trusting the net will appear if you need it. You can't sit back and wait for the new you to emerge like a butterfly from a cocoon. You might well continue to live some kind of a life safe inside your cocoon; you might even see the sun rise every day, but you might never again fully appreciate it.

Creating a day worth living:
Get up early, express gratitude for what you have.
Do something productive. Do something fun. Do
something for someone else. Get some sunlight.
Exercise—it doesn't matter what—just do some
exercise. Put a smile on someone's face. Express
gratitude or compliment someone. Learn or
do something new. That's it—Now, wasn't that
better!! — cornercanyoncounseling.com

Chapter Three

ONE YEAR ANNIVERSARY TRIP

O ne year after Tony passed away I indulged myself in what would turn out to be a life changing experience. It came about very accidentally.

It all began in April of 2016 when Krista, my very dear friend and yoga teacher, invited me to a Qigong Healing Forum presented by teacher Jeff Primack in Daytona Beach. I had never heard of Qigong, but since it was close to home and I could sleep in my own bed every night, I decided to check it out. I have always respected and appreciated Krista's judgment. She knew I was going through an adjustment and grieving process after the loss of my husband and felt it might be something that would be helpful to me.

So I did a little research and learned Qigong has roots in Chinese medicine, philosophy, and martial arts. and is traditionally viewed as a practice to cultivate and balance chi, translated as "life energy."

This certainly piqued my interest—enough for me to register for the weekend forum. And believe me when I say that I was not disappointed. The forum ranged wide and deep into how we can best balance our life energy. It was not only about physical and mental exercise, it also covered nutrition, healthy eating, and the importance of breathing. We learned about red pepper paste and smoothies, and I'll share those recipes with you later.

FINDING A NEW SPIRITUAL CONNECTION IN HAWAII

Throughout the weekend I felt sure I was taking on good fuel for my healing journey. I was moving forward, and had the weekend been the end of it, I would have felt satisfied. However, as if on cue, I learned that Jeff was offering a seven-day Qigong retreat in Hawaii in June. Luck, or divine providence, continued to shape the moment when I realized I was already planning a trip to California to visit my aunt in San Diego the week before the retreat was to begin. It was a like a bolt of lightning hit me when I realized the synchronicity of this retreat with my already scheduled trip to California.

Yes, my expectations were very high after the growth I'd experienced in one weekend.

So I meditated during the weekend of the Daytona Beach forum about registering for the retreat in Hawaii. I am at heart a practical person—which is perhaps why I chose astrology as a path—but it certainly felt like this was divine providence, like something I was destined to do. And after all, I kept reminding myself, I would already be half way to Hawaii when I was in California.

When I studied my astrology chart for the dates of the Hawaii retreat I saw that all of the stars were aligned and it was exactly what I needed to do. I felt that this trip would be a major part of my "healing journey" and I would return home different, more evolved, with a mended soul.

For those who speak astrology, you will understand why this was such an opportune time for me. For those who don't, please accept that it was. I realized that the transiting moon was going to be in the sign of Aries conjunct my sun in Aries on the day the retreat was to begin. I knew that the timing was perfect. This was like having my very own personal new moon, which is a perfect time to begin something new and make a fresh start. In addition to that, transiting Mars was making a connection to my natal Jupiter. Mars the motivator and Jupiter is the guardian angel and expander. When Jupiter is activated by Mars it is a very favorable time for traveling or launching any new project. It is basically known as a "lucky time."

* * *

I was still feeling the amazing impact the conference in Daytona Beach had on my life, so I could only imagine what a week at a retreat in Hawaii would do for me—and at this moment *me* had to be my focus. I was still practicing as an astrologer and helping other people with the challenges in their lives while I was healing and adjusting to the loss of my husband. I felt that I needed to take this opportunity to work solely on myself and regain my inner peace and strength. Yes, my expectations were very high after the growth I experienced in one weekend. Now bear in mind that I did not know a single soul who was planning to attend this retreat, except for Jeff, the instructor, but that fact didn't frighten me. I was being drawn to Hawaii almost thoughtlessly, like sailors drawn in by the song of a sea nymph. I knew instinctively that the call I was hearing was genuine. And believe me when I say that I was not disappointed.

With all the pieces synchronizing naturally, the decision to go to Hawaii was simple. All I had to do was say yes. The siren song of the big island of Hawaii was calling, but there was one more factor: the retreat, just a few months off now, was in June— the one year anniversary of my husband's passing. I have a beautiful condo on the ocean but I had no desire to be there at that this time.

I was planning to fly home from California the exact same day the retreat was to begin, so still feeling a Qigong afterglow, I moved quickly and changed my travel plans.

It was Monday June 27th, 2016. I was so excited; I couldn't believe the day had actually come. Still, as the dream was finally unfolding, I suddenly experienced mixed emotions about this adventure. Although I had lived on Oahu in my youth when my father was stationed in the Navy, I had never been to the Big Island of Hawaii. This was going to be a

---

totally new territory and experience for me.

My fears were soon overcome by the joy and optimism I felt as the last few days ticked away. I wanted to soar and enjoy each and every experience of this "retreat." For those who speak the language and want to follow the endnote to the back of the book, please do. You will appreciate everything that was going on in my chart the day I arrived on the Island. For others, let's just say all my ducks were lining up—that is, very supportive astrologically speaking. You might not be surprised to hear I actually studied my chart for this trip before I made the commitment. I knew from what I saw this would be an exciting, life changing experience—the trip of a lifetime. I had believed that from the moment I first heard about it. I was excited and ready for the unknown adventure, but I had to know what my chart said.

I had read Elizabeth Gilbert's book *Eat, Pray, Love*. I even saw the movie, several times, which totally captured my emotions. So when I embarked on this Hawaiian Retreat adventure I was excited. I wasn't expecting to find the "love" part of the book, but I did have very strong Jupiter/Mars connections going on, which could indicate a romantic connection. At the very least it was going to be a wonderful adventure, which is what it turned out to be. So as it turned out, for my one year anniversary of Tony's passing I had chosen to begin with pray, not eat or love, which is why I chose this Qigong retreat.

I was in very good spirits as I embarked for the San Diego airport on what I felt certain would be a spiritual journey. I knew in my heart this was going to be an amazing week. It was going to help me rediscover the light within me so I could appreciate and honor it. I felt fortunate and blessed to be able to do this at this time in my life. I began to feel the serenity and calmness as I started to do the Qigong breathing exercises as a part of my daily routine. What I didn't know was how much hard work it was going to be.

The first day . . . Upon arriving on the Big Island I was overwhelmed by its beauty. I didn't realize it was an agricultural island. The retreat compound where I stayed was on the Kona side of the island, also known as the rainy side. We were very fortunate that it mostly rained only at night during our retreat.

When I landed at the little Kona airport I felt like I had entered another word or dimension in time. Jeff Primack, the Qigong instructor, was also our chauffeur and tour guide and made our first introductions to what appeared to be a very unpopulated and beautiful emerald in the middle of the Pacific.

I will confess that for a moment I wanted to run.

This was certainly very different from when I had lived in Hawaii as a child with my family when my father was in the Navy stationed on Oahu. We had lived on Waikiki, which even at that time was much more populated than the Big Island. This was totally new territory and a new experience for me.

The drive up the mountain to the compound was amazingly beautiful. I had absolutely no comprehension of the beauty and experiences that I was going to encounter over the next week. I knew there would be no electricity and that "the facilities" were the outdoor variety. It was sort of like camping with running water.

There was no air conditioning, but there always seemed to be a nice island breeze and it rained a part of every day, so I never felt hot. In fact it was actually cool in the evenings when the sun went down. The outdoor shower stalls had running hot and cold water and were located across a field about 100 yards from my cabin. Right next to them were two community sinks for brushing your teeth and washing your hands. The outdoor flushing toilet stalls were about 100 yards in the opposite direction. So I got lots of exercise. And even though I didn't need to, I did lose weight.

The modest, sparsely furnished two-person cabins had very comfortable posturepedic mattresses. I slept like a baby every night. The open air screening allowed the tropical breeze to cool the evening air.

There are no words to describe the quiet and isolated feeling of this compound. It was surrounded by natural running streams and beautiful waterfalls. It was like nothing I had ever seen or experienced before. I felt like I was in a movie. I felt surrounded by God and angels. But it was a huge adjustment. I did not have a roommate. No electricity, no computer, no cell phone, no TV, no internet and NO WINE. What was a person to do?

I will confess that for a moment when I first arrived and saw the facilities I wanted to run, to fly back to civilization in California, but instead I focused on centering myself, on seeing the upside to being free from our devises. This was truly going to be a spiritual, healing time with no distractions. It was as close to connecting with nature as I had ever been. The evening sky was like a field of diamonds with no electric lights or emissions to mask its beauty. The moon was in the last quarter of its waning phase, so there was not much in the way of light of the moon to compete with the dark of the night.

It was truly a paradise retreat with the exception of the deep emotional work that lay ahead of me.

We were told during our orientation meeting that coffee and papaya would be available in the dome, which was a picturesque walk across a green field. The kitchen was also there with a generator that provided the only electricity in the compound. The outdoor bathroom facility, which did flush, was on the way. Our morning breathing and Qigong practice would begin at 8 a.m. in an outdoor covered pavilion overlooking a spectacular running stream which fed into a waterfall. This was truly God's country. There is no other way to describe it.

We met the staff and our fellow journeyers during this first gathering in the dome. I was very surprised to learn that all of the participants' had traveled to Hawaii from Florida. Here I was 5,000 miles from home meeting people who lived only 60 miles from me.

After coffee and papaya we walked to the open air pavilion overlooking the mountain stream and got right to work. Jeff led us into a Qigong breathing exercise. It was so powerful and intense that it brought out an overflow of emotions in me. Unspoken prayer was pouring out of my heart. It was intense to say the least. At that moment I knew my life-changing quest had begun in earnest.

It wasn't all smooth and easy. It took me several days to decompress and recompose from the high drive, high gear activities that I was used to in my daily life. After my husband passed away the previous year I went into overdrive. In my true Arian nature, my survival mode was to stay busy. Every sun sign has its way of coping and that was mine. So this retreat was totally a foreign path for me. No connection to the outside world. Was this to become my new reality? Really? Would I be able to achieve and maintain a sense of peace and acceptance within myself without exterior distractions and stimulations? I gave myself over, allowing the retreat's benefits in, rather than resisting them.

In addition to the physical and mental healing benefits of this retreat, I learned a great deal about the benefits our instructor Jeff Primack describes in his book, *Food—Healing Cooking with Qi.*

Each morning when we first got up we were offered a variation of a fresh healthy smoothie, or half of a papaya, and coffee or tea. After our Qigong practice which usually took anywhere between an hour or two we enjoyed our choice of a healthy omelet with a variation of fresh vegetables and/or goat cheese. Asparagus was my favorite and of course the home made pepper paste which I have continued to make and share with my friends and neighbors. Some mornings we even had little fresh langostinos also known as baby lobsters that Jeff had caught in his mountain stream traps. I knew I wouldn't recall every delicious meal and desert, so I purchased Jeff's cookbook, and his smoothie book, *Smoothie Formulas*, which includes 95 delicious high-photochemical recipes.

My morning smoothie became a major part of

---

my healing journey when I returned home. I have continued to enjoy making the "Anti-Inflammation Smoothie" for pain and arthritis.

RECIPE FOR "ANTI-INFLAMMATION SMOOTHIE"

2 c. distilled water

30 cherries, remove pits

1/2 organic cucumber

3 wedges papaya, no seeds.

1 inch ginger root

1 inch turmeric root

1 inch thick pineapple ring

1 pineapple stem

I tend to use a little more ginger and turmeric root then the recipe calls for and fewer cherries. I make this in a NutriBullet and divide it into two portions. I believe this has helped my arthritis and improved my energy level, and it's wonderful for the digestive system.

After a healthy, delicious breakfast Jeff would lead us on a spectacular hike or walk through the lush, tropical wooded fields covered with moss and ferns. Those who were more adventurous and sure-footed also explored the rock embedded streams where the water was constantly flowing.

I personally found it more with in my comfort zone to stay on dry ground where I felt more secure. I certainly did not want to be evacuated back to the mainland in an air ambulance. I knew my limitations and I wasn't there to prove anything. I was there to find myself and redefine myself.

GOING WITHIN TO FIND PEACE AND HAPPINESS

As I was coming to the end of this week of hard work, isolation, meditation, and transformation, I started thinking about how I was going to integrate this feeling of peacefulness into my daily life. I came to the conclusion that only I could make myself happy. I needed to internalize the experience and make it part of my biology, so I could go within naturally and without conscious manipulation to find peace and my personal happiness.

As the week wound down, I kept reminding myself that I was fortunate and blessed to have been able to make this journey. I wanted to savor every minute and enjoy the beauty of the tropical, mystical paradise. And I wanted to take home with me everything I had learned, everything I was feeling.

What changes did the Qigong retreat help create in me?

- More energy and mental clarity
- Better balance
- Better focus and concentration
- A feeling of calmness
- More patience
- Better nutrition and food education

I discovered that stress makes you tired. I was amazed that I wasn't ever really tired the entire time that I was there.

And as an added bonus, it even helped my golf game when I got back home by slowing down my backswing!

In fact, my new practice of Qigong helped open many doors for me. I grew healthier in body, mind, and spirit. It was an education in nutrition. It improved my physical movement and exercise practice. It gave me more energy as I learned breathing exercises to reach a deeper meditative state.

There were physiological benefits like improving my blood circulation, lowering my blood pressure, and the removal of dioxins from my body.

When I returned from Hawaii I knew I was ready to begin on my second book. I had found the inner peace I needed. I now could look inside without as much fear. Sure it was difficult, but I no longer shied away from the reality.

WRITING FEEDS MY SOUL . . .

I have learned over the years that writing feeds my soul and after my week in Hawaii my soul was in a feeding frenzy—calm but energized. Writing my daily posts on my *AstrologyTalk* Facebook page, my monthly Astrology Newsletter, my journal all feed my soul. The challenge, I told myself, was to find or make time to write another book.

I guess it wasn't until I really got motivated and felt that I had something to share again, something to say that could help others through their healing journey, that I made the commitment to myself to focus on this book. My one year anniversary trip helped take me to that place.

What drives your engine? What are you passionate about? What motivates you to get out of bed and get moving in the morning? These are all thought provoking subjects that Elizabeth Gilbert brought out in *Big Magic, Creative Living Beyond Fear*.

Do you find solace or enjoyment in music, cooking, entertaining friends, reading or watching TV? I know one of the things I really missed was cooking after my husband passed away. He always loved my cooking, never complained and was easy to please.

I missed watching, golf, football, tennis and our favorite shows together. It took a long time before I could watch any of the things we used to watch together. I couldn't even cook a meal without crying.

LIFE IS ABOUT CHANGE

If there is one thing that I have learned over the years, it is that "life is about change." Nothing remains the same. I guess the big question is how do we deal with change in our life. How do we survive change. How do we move beyond survival and prosper—perhaps in ways we never imagined.

I did eventually begin to watch football, golf and tennis again, but of course it wasn't the same without him. I started cooking again and inviting friends in for dinner. I still love to entertain but of course that's not the same without him either. But then, nothing remains the same. Every sunrise and every sunset are different, beautiful in their own way, each casting different shades of red, yellow, and blue. In the same way, each of our days is different.

My dear friend Krista just happened to give me Elizabeth Gilbert's book for my birthday. And she also started the chain reaction that led to me studying Qigong in Hawaii. It seems as with everything that Krista does, her timing is perfect. If we are to move smoothly through this life timing is everything.

My first book was published in 2011 when Jupiter was traveling through my 9th house, conjunct my Sun which is the house that rules publications. I knew when I was in Hawaii that Jupiter was going to be traveling through my 3rd house from September of 2016 until October of 2017. Since the 3rd house rules writing and communications, I knew that if I was going to write another book that would be the ideal time to do it. So everything was in my favor—time to get to work!

> *"Shoot for the moon and if you miss,*
> *you will still be among the stars."*
> — Les Brown

Chapter Four

SHOW ME THE GLINT OF THE MOON

Not long after returning from Hawaii I planned a trip to Milwaukee, where I would visit with Betty Riley, the remarkable woman who years earlier had led me into astrology. I wasn't consciously thinking *I'll return to my roots so I can better remember who I am while traveling toward my new normal.* I wasn't thinking it, but it turned out to be true.

As I was packing, I began considering which books to take along. I always like to carry a few books to read on the plane. Although I have a Kindle, I'm not very good about downloading my books, so I try to select books from my library that don't take much space in my backpack. I came across a book called *The Astrologer's Node Book,* by Donna Van Toen, which was published in 1981—probably the same year I bought it. I could see that I must have read it before because I had highlighted paragraphs. But for the life me I didn't remember reading it.

ANOTHER TOOL TO AID IN THE HEALING JOURNEY, THROUGH THE EYES OF AN ASTROLOGER . . .

Again, as God or luck would have it, it was exactly what I needed to be reading at the time and on that trip. I have always found the lunar cycle to be extremely helpful in my personal life and in working with my clients. And I have always been aware of the lunar nodes. The moon's nodes, also known as the lunar nodes, are imaginary points that mark off a sort of celestial equator. They are used by astronomers in the calculation of astronomical distances, eclipses and other important data.

Although the moon and its nodes are not planets, they do play an important role in our astrological chart. If you do not speak the language and this is new to you, please indulge me while I take a side step and share my passion for astrology with you in an area that's not as mainstream as knowing your sun sign. If you've never followed astrology at all, you might discover why so many people enjoy mixing it into their philosophy of life.

The South Node: Revealing Past Lives, Natural Abilities

The South Node reveals the gifts that you bring into this lifetime, your sweet spot, your comfort zone. You will be innately good in these areas of life, and may begin your early path based on your South Node leanings. While this can bring a sense of satisfaction, it is unlikely to elevate you to "Blissville." There's a sense of "been there, done that" in the field of South Node activities—a feeling of déjà vu. The key is to use your South Node as a springboard into your North Node destiny, much like a foreigner living abroad

46   Kelly Lowe

will always feel most comfortable speaking her native language, even if she's lived in her new country for many years. The South Node in your horoscope is your hometown, perhaps not the place you want to settle permanently, but somewhere cozy to visit when you need to feel a sense of place or belonging.

The North Node: Your Destiny That's Calling

The North Node is the exact opposite zodiac sign of the South Node. It illuminates the terrain that's calling your name, but climbing to the peak of this mountain is like trekking up Mt. Everest. You'll have to lighten up your baggage and enlist a proverbial Sherpa to get you up that hill. It's your learning curve.

... it was like a bolt of lightning struck me!

North Node activities require you to stretch out of your comfort zone. Once you do, you'll be amazed by how fulfilled you feel. It's like the activation of your life's mission. The sooner you align yourself with this path, the more purpose-driven your life will become. However, you will often return to your South Node as that "ace in the hole"—kind of like returning home to your roots, even after you've made your way in the world. It is your innate comfort zone.

As I was re-reading Donna Van Toen's book on the plane, it was like a bolt of lightning struck me! The person sitting next to me even asked me if I was okay when she saw the expressions on my face. It answered so many questions for me and in my mind opened so many new doors. This information was there all of the time for me, but until I was ready to receive it, it didn't appear.

It reminds me of the saying, "When the student

is ready the teacher will appear." So I will be using this tool along with the lunar cycles in my healing journey and interpreting it when working with my clients.

THE MANY FACES OF THE MOON

Following the lunar cycle is perhaps my favorite and most reliable astrological timing tool. As the Moon travels from new to full it can be a tremendous aid for planning and timing events. The lunar and solar eclipses are especially "event significant." The lunar cycle can give you a tremendous edge in your professional and personal life. It is without a doubt one of the major factors that is available in timing events to achieve your desired results.

The moon is about our emotions and how we feel. It affects how we react to emotional situations. It is also a great aid to help us get in touch with and understand our emotions. I found it to be especially helpful as I was going through my healing journey. For example when I knew we were approaching a full moon I knew that my emotions would be running rampant as if on steroids. I would find myself crying more and overreacting to my emotions. But then I would take a few deep breaths and remind myself that these feelings would pass. I also found meditation, Qigong, yoga, and exercise to be helpful.

YOUR PERSONAL GPS

Following the lunar cycle each month is like having your own personal GPS for your journey through life. The lunar cycle can be used in timing your activities and is one of the most valuable tools you can use. In many Eastern countries, timing by the planets is so important that practically no event takes place without first setting up an astrological chart. Many times weddings take place in the middle of the night because that is when the planetary influences are the most favorable.

Since ancient times the cycle of the Moon from new to full to new has been observed and correlated with events on Earth. The early farmers learned that sowing seed at the New Moon leads to better harvest. Sailors learned to time their travels by the phase of the Moon, which everyone knows controls the tides. In addition to controlling the tides, the Moon rules the ebb and flow of the bodily fluids, emotions, feelings and state of mind.

FISHING AND THE MOON

Living at the ocean has given me first-hand knowledge of the trends of the fishing boats during the fishing season. Saltwater fishing is an occupation—or hobby—with a lot of self-anointed "experts" who often disagree with each other on just about everything, but catch records of professionals, recreational anglers and scientific studies say that saltwater species are more active for four days leading up to the Full Moon and for four days after the New Moon. There are other variables to consider, like water temperature and time of day, but when the Moon is full the trolling fishing boats light up the horizon like a Christmas tree. The tides are noticeably higher during the new and full phases of the Moon and the increased movement of water may hold the explanation for why the fish seem more active at this time.

STORM PATTERNS

At the New Moon, the Sun and Moon are together in the heavens creating a massive concentration of energy, which can lead to the development of strong storm systems. This can be an emotional storm or a full blown hurricane. Think about how you feel when there is a Full Moon. Energy levels tend to run higher, less sleep is needed. The New Moon is the time to plant the seeds that you will harvest during the Full Moon.

Although the New Moon and the Full Moon and the few days leading up to them are the strongest times in the cycle, the total lunar cycle needs to be taken into consideration when timing an event or project. As I mentioned earlier, following the lunar cycle each month can be just like having a personal GPS to help you with your journey through life. It is a day-to-day guide for planning your actions, and paying close attention to it will help you to better achieve your desired goals. Eclipse cycles can also add a strong impact on the weather, but that's the subject of my next chapter.

You will want to pay special attention if there is a storm approaching during a New or Full Moon. A perfect example that comes to mind is the series of hurricanes that hit Florida in 2004. I can still recall the weather forecast for the approaching storm as I was observing its daily movement in relation to the lunar cycle. We were approaching the New Moon of August 16 when Hurricane Charley, having come ashore on Florida's West Coast a little south of Tampa, was predicted to travel across the state and hit the East Coast of Florida.

We pulled down the shutters on our condo and battened down the hatches for what proved to be a thrashing, nightmare of a storm. In the pitch black of the night we could hear the shrieking sounds as the eye of the storm reached us and rushed over us. It has been said so often but it's true: it sounded like a fast moving train rolling over our head. We were one of the few residents in the building who chose to stay and weather the storm.

I had survived Karen, a 210 knot typhoon when I lived on Guam, an island in the Pacific, while my father was stationed there in the Navy. I wasn't about to be chased out of my home by a hurricane that may or may not come our way. But it certainly did come our way. It was a doozy. Everyone in our building who did not have hurricane shutters lost their windows and sliding glass doors. Their interiors were left in shambles. All of the condo units located under these vulnerable units were also flooded as the water made its way through the ceilings and walls.

It seems that the condominium building located next to ours had a flat pebble roof and the pebbles where jetted through the air like bullets, destroying every window pane that was not covered. Fortunately, our shutters saved us. Fortunately, our neighbors above us also had shutters which prevented us from being flooded from above. We were one of the few units that did not suffer water damage. Our storm shutters looked like they had been riveted with buckshot.

When we poked our heads out the door after the storm moved on, the parking lot looked like a war zone. There was furniture, debris and glass everywhere. It felt like we were in a bombed out, evacuated city and we were the only living souls around. It was devastating and brought back my childhood memories of typhoon Karen. In addition to the structural damage of the storm, the erosion of the shoreline was disastrous and heartbreaking.

Just three weeks later on September 8, 2004, hurricane Frances was forecast to be heading our way. Of course we thought, no way, not again. When it seemed that "again" really was going to happen, I referred to my astrological calendar. This time the storm was six days prior to the September 14 New Moon, so I figured it would not be as devastating. We chose to stay, battening down the hatches once again. The biggest problem was that people had not had time to repair their roofs from the last hurricane and the water had not had time to seep into the ground. Unfortunately, the already damaged shoreline was getting another unneeded beating.

As if that were not enough, on September 26, 2004, hurricane Jeanne struck us. The Full Moon was September 28. She alone was not as destructive as hurricanes Charley and Frances, but she certainly added to the already disastrous situation. There was already way too much water and not enough time to repair roofs in between these lunar cycles. Of course, it goes without saying that we—and most of our neighboring communities—were without electricity for days or weeks. Some people didn't even get their electric turned back on before the next storm hit.

The lesson to this story is that you may want to consider evacuating if there is a major storm predicted to be heading your way around the time of a Full or New Moon. You can't stop it but you can get out of its way.

Hurricanes are stressful enough when you have a partner to weather them with, but when the person with whom you had already weathered three storms is no longer with you, it's even more dramatic. Yes, with Hurricane Matthew approaching I guess I could have packed up and gone to Orlando and stayed with my son, but I decided to stay at the beach and weather it out with my neighbors.

Hurricane Matthew paid his visit in October of 2016. Fortunately, it was not a direct hit to our immediate area. As I was tracking its progress I wasn't too concerned since I knew it was not a full or new moon.

YOUR LUNAR GPS:
A NAVIGATION TOOL TO HELP YOU IN YOUR DAILY LIFE

I feel that I would be remiss if I did not share this information with you. You can easily learn to use the cycles of the Moon to help plan your activities so that you can enjoy optimum results. Most calendars provide this information. Of course, astrological calendars provide more in-depth information.

New Moon – When the Moon is traveling 0-45 degrees ahead of the Sun it is considered to be in its new phase. This is an excellent time to begin anything that you would want to have longevity. It is considered to be the germination cycle. This is an excellent time for putting ideas into action by initiating and outwardly directing your activities.

There is a direct correlation between what is already happening in your life and how you will feel and react to the energy of the New Moon. You may enjoy feelings of rest and peace if all is going well; or chaos, disorganization and confusion if your life is already in turmoil. Whichever is the case, whatever you initiate during this cycle should be fruitful. Just be careful. If you choose to do something harmful—for example, to initiate a campaign of revenge against someone—it may get out of hand. If you choose to begin a positive endeavor, it is likely to blossom. I chose this cycle to begin writing this book.

It is best to avoid elective surgery during this phase of the Moon, as there will tend to be more bleeding.

First Quarter or Waxing Moon – (seven days following the New Moon) When the Moon is 90-135 degrees ahead of the Sun it is still considered to be in the growth and development phase and activities that apply to the New Moon cycle also apply to the Waxing Moon.

Second Quarter – When the Moon is approximately 140–175 degrees ahead of the Sun the energy and activity is a continuation of the 1st quarter activities.

Third Quarter or Full Moon – (fourteen days following the New Moon) When the Moon is 180 degrees from the Sun it is considered to be in its maturity or fruition phase. This is when you will see the fruits of your labor and the seeds that you have planted during a New Moon cycle come to fruition. Emotions tend to run high. Depending upon what is going on in your life, you may feel ecstatic or depressed. Feelings and emotions tend to be exaggerated when the Moon is full. Elective surgery should also be avoided during this phase of the Moon as there tends to be more bleeding and swelling.

It has been my experience that people often times require less sleep or have difficulty sleeping a couple of nights before the Full Moon. Since energy levels tend to be higher, this is an excellent time to escalate your exercise program. You should be able to accomplish a great deal during this lunar cycle

Fourth Quarter or Waning Moon – (seven days following the Full Moon) When the Moon is traveling 90–135 degrees behind the Sun it is in its disintegration and drawing back phase. This is the time for reorganization, rest and reflection. This is when you will want to step back and get the big picture, to regroup and analyze your progress with initiatives you have already begun.

Balsamic Moon or Dark of the Moon – (fourteen days following the Full Moon) This is the 24-hour period just before the New Moon. During this phase of the Moon the Sun's light is not reflective. It is *not* a good time to initiate any projects that you would want to produce long-term results. This is also *not* the best time to be making new contacts, especially if you happen to work in the field of sales or marketing. This is also not the preferred time to sign contracts or legal documents as there may be a lack of clarity, or an inability to follow through.

This should be a quiet, working behind the scenes time. It is best to avoid high expectations, major decisions or physical projects. You will want to focus on mental tasks for the best use of your time on these days. This is a great time to plan and prepare for what you want to do when the Moon is new. Energy levels tend to run low during this cycle, so it's better not to push yourself.

THE MOON TRAVELING THROUGH THE SUN SIGNS

This is another tool that can be used to help you plan your activities in order to achieve a result that you'll appreciate.

I have found it to be very helpful to pay attention to the sign that the Moon is traveling through each day, as this can be a tremendous aid in helping you plan your activities. For example, when the Moon is in the sign of Virgo it is an excellent time for activities that require attention to details.

Since it takes the Moon two and a half days to travel through each Sun sign there is ample time for all activities in the course of a month. The Moon's movement through each of its signs can be followed easily with an astrological calendar.

It is also important to note on an astrological calendar that period of time when the Moon is *void of course*. The Moon is V/C (*void of course*) when it makes its last major aspect with another planet before going into the next sign. An aspect is the same as a connection to another planet. For example, the planet may be in the same degree and sign as the Moon or even opposite the Moon. It remains *void of course* until it enters a new sign, in which it will make another aspect. An astrological aspect refers to the relationship or connection between the planets.

During the V/C period it is advisable not to make any major decisions or sign contracts. It would be best not to start anything that you want to be long lasting. Think of it as a balsamic or dark of the Moon cycle. This can last for as little as a few minutes or up to several hours. Again, an astrological calendar will be instrumental in helping you chart your course.

It has been my experience that when the Moon is *void of course* it is very difficult to bring anything to completion, or even accomplish something as simple as reaching someone on the phone.

Observing the Moon as it travels from one sign to the next is like reading your personal barometer and acting accordingly. A barometer measures the barometric pressure in the atmosphere. It lets us know when the pressure is dropping and therefore rain is forthcoming. With that knowledge you can plan your activities more effectively. You probably would not want to schedule a picnic when the barometer is dropping. In the same way, as the Moon is traveling through each sign you can take advantage by timing your activities as they relate to the sign and task at hand.

When the Moon Reaches Your Sun Sign . . .

When the Moon is traveling through the sign of **Aries** it is an excellent time to be an initiator. It is a positive time to start a new job or project. This is especially true when a New Moon is in Aries, but be careful—tempers tend to run hot and patience can be short. I would suggest not doing anything that might create confrontation. I've noticed that drivers tend to be more aggressive and impatient during this lunar cycle.

When the Moon is traveling through the sign of **Taurus** you will find your focus and attention drawn toward reinforcing your values and sense of security. You may spend this time balancing your checkbook or paying bills. You will want to evaluate what is really important to you. This is a good time to begin anything that you want to have longevity. For example, open a new savings account or start a new business venture. It is also a wonderful time to plant a garden, especially if it is a New Moon.

When the Moon is traveling through the sign of **Gemini** you will be drawn toward mental and expressive activities. You may find yourself drawn to reading, writing, exploring new areas of knowledge, and wanting to communicate more. You may also have a sudden wish to take a short trip, or just to get yourself in motion by running errands around town. Your desire is to expand your horizons, but you will need to prioritize because there is a tendency to become scattered.

When the Moon is in the sign of **Cancer** it is in its comfortable placement. This is a perfect time for nurturing. You will be more interested in domestic activities, particularly if your natal Sun or Moon is in the sign of Cancer. You will be drawn to spending more time at home and taking care of family matters. Don't be surprised if you feel an impulse to spend time in your kitchen trying out some new recipes.

The period when the Moon is in **Leo** is a time to let the child in you come out and play. You will want to be artistic, romantic and creative. You will enjoy going to a movie, a play, a concert, or out to dinner. This could be a good time to play the lottery or go to Las Vegas, especially if other aspects in your chart are set up well to support this.

When the Moon is in the sign of **Virgo** it is a great time to get organized—particularly if Mercury is retrograde. You will feel motivated to take care of details, like cleaning out closets and drawers and your desk. You will want to take care of health matters such as doctor's appointments, health checkups and physicals. If it happens to be a "new" Moon in Virgo it is a great time to begin a diet or exercise program.

When the Moon is in the sign of **Libra** it is an excellent time for negotiating and dealing with others on a one-to-one basis. For instance, you are likely to have that heart-to-heart talk you have been putting off with your spouse or co-worker. Since this is typically a non-confrontational time, the outcome should be fruitful. This can be a time to enjoy the peace and harmony you have been seeking in your life.

The Moon in the sign of **Scorpio** can be a very strong emotional time. This is not a good time for confrontation, especially if it is a Full Moon. People often feel secretive or less communicative during this cycle. It is a good time for regenerative actions and investigative work. You can get to the bottom of things, and loose ends dangling in the back of your mind can finally be tied off. Insurance questions, or legal matters like a will, may need to be taken care of. This is a good time to do so.

When the Moon is in the sign of **Sagittarius** it is a good time for spiritual development and philosophical thought. You may be motivated to enroll in a college course, or to continue or start a new line of study. This is a great time to begin a long trip or vacation. People tend to feel upbeat and optimistic during this cycle. It is a good time to open yourself up without apprehension or prior expectations and see what flows in.

The Moon in the sign of **Capricorn** is a good time to become organized and bring structure into your life. People tend to be more critical during this cycle. This is the time that you will want to take care of business. It is a no-nonsense time. Your time is better spent working than playing.

When the Moon is in the sign of **Aquarius** it is an excellent time for socializing, particularly if Venus is making a favorable aspect in your chart. It is great for attending club or organization activities, and parties. There is a tendency to be more creative and open minded during this cycle.

The Moon in the sign of **Pisces** is a good time for enhancing spiritual development. You will want to get in touch with your inner emotions. People will tend to be more compassionate and in tune to other people's feelings. There is also a tendency to have your feelings hurt more easily, especially if your natal Sun or Moon is in this sign.

It is especially important to observe the sign that the Moon is in when there is an eclipse, as this magnifies the activities and makes them even more significant.

"Healing comes from taking responsibility: to realize that it is you, and no one else, who creates your thoughts, your feelings, and your actions." — Peter Sheperd

Chapter Five

THANK YOU ELIZABETH GILBERT

J ust as every tree needs its seed, I believe every writer needs inspiration.

I believe that Elizabeth was my seed, inspiration, and motivation. *Eat Pray Love* gave me the idea and desire to register for my retreat across the Pacific. Although the "Big Island of Hawaii" was an exciting and beautiful place to visit, and I was open to new horizons in my life, it was scary to think about embarking on a week-long adventure where I would not know a single soul except for the instructor.

As I wrote earlier, the trip turned out to be all I desired but even after I arrived at the retreat I continued to feel strong doubts and wanted to run from this new thing. Because I came to understand that great things often have costs, but paying that price turns out to be part of the prize you receive.

My trip to Hawaii was so crucial that I'll risk repeating some of what I said before to tell you more about why it changed me. I've heard of people traveling joyfully to India to meditate at the base of the Himalayas and invite enlightenment into their lives, which they claimed to have found. It all sounded too easy. I went to Hawaii with great trepidation and anticipation. When I arrived at the Kona Airport I looked around for Jeff the Qigong leader and volunteer chauffer. It was a very small airport so I didn't have to wait very long, but there was a moment when I thought, what if no one shows up? What if I can't find him?

I did have his cell number, which I called and left a message. As it turned out there were two other women also waiting to be picked up. So we had a very enjoyable visit on the drive up the mountain to the retreat compound, which was beautiful. Meeting new people helped me relax and find a temporary escape from feeling alone.

There was an immediate sense of relief when I saw Jeff and climbed into his SUV. The front seat was full of wonderful island fruits and vegetables which I looked forward to experiencing. And I must say I was not disappointed with his chef's presentations.

When the two other women and I climbed into the SUV together there was an immediate connection, even though I had never laid eyes on them before. I could feel they were in Hawaii seeking their own version of what I was there for. We often meet people in life who are at points on their journey that are different from ours, but when we sense we are all moving in the same direction we know we share the same soul. This was indeed going to be a special week.

I quickly learned that Maya and Lee were also from Florida and they were planning to be married on the Big Island after the retreat. As it turned out, I became friends with them and I was invited to their wedding. I actually was their wedding photographer. I couldn't believe that I flew across the Pacific to meet people who lived only 150 miles from me.

As we entered the compound I was filled with awe at the natural beauty, open land and isolation. I was also overwhelmed by the feeling of isolation. There were twelve of us who had signed up for this once in a life time experience, but I was alone. I was not used to traveling alone. What in God's earth ever made me decided to do this.

> Being alone was one of the most difficult things I had to adjust to.

I couldn't help thinking about the Hawaiian golfing vacation that Tony and I had planned years ago and had to cancel when my father was diagnosed with lung cancer. So this was a bittersweet trip. This was meant to be a healing trip. But was I ready for it?

My very first thought was to turn around and get on the next plane back to my aunt's house in San Diego, which was familiar to me. There I would feel safe and comfortable. Since we had limited cell service and limited power to recharge our phones, I was restricted in the calls I could make. But the first call I made was to my aunt to ask her if she could check on flights back to California for me.

Fortunately for me, they were very expensive and limited, so I was forced to stay on this beautiful paradise island for seven days "alone." I was someone who was used to being busy all the time, watching TV, emailing, internet connections, texting, calling friends, and having a couple of glasses of wine in the evening. This was all part of my routine. This would all change for the next seven days.

Once I gave in to my fate, it took me most of the first two days to decompress and appreciate what I was about to experience. I kept thinking about Elizabeth Gilbert when she was scrubbing the floors at the Ashram in India and sitting for hours in meditation in total stillness and silence. Yes, we also had quiet time at our retreat. And anyone who knows me, knows that I am not a quiet person. I love to socialize, and after my husband passed away I hated being alone.

Being alone was one of the most difficult things I had to adjust to. I was used to my husband being around almost all of the time, especially when he was so sick in the last few years before his passing—which was one of the many reasons I felt such a void in my life.

And now, here I was all alone in my cabin with a bunk bed and nothing else. Since the retreat was not full I didn't have a cabin mate. I was left to my own space and my own thoughts except for the scheduled activities.

As it turned out one of the scheduled activities was hiking through lush, hilly tropical fields and across bubbling streams. Although the tropical fields were doable for me, I opted out because of the river streams. I didn't want to take a chance on reinjuring my quadricep tendon which had been repaired with major surgery a couple years prior to my husband's passing. It had been a very long healing and recovery process, and I certainly didn't want to take any unnecessary risks while so far from home.

And then there was the total hip replacement that I had two months after Tony's passing. No, I couldn't be hiking through any slippery mountain streams on this trip. So when everyone else went off on their hikes, I was alone at the compound with more time to meditate and think. It was a cram course in being alone.

It was now two weeks past the one year anniversary of Tony's death and I was thinking that I should be feeling a lot better than I was about being alone. So I used the time to "go inside," to meditate and pray. I've always heard that praying is talking to God and meditating is when you listen to him. At home, before leaving on this retreat, I was neither talking or listening. Believe me, I wanted to, even though I knew it could lead me into places I was avoiding. That could have been it—avoidance. Despite living alone I could always find some distraction—TV, phones, internet, anything—to keep me from meditating. I just was not able to quite my mind when I was home alone.

It reminded me of that movie "Home Alone" where eight-year-old, Macaulay Culkin, gets really busy and into all kinds of trouble when his parents left him home alone. It's not that I was looking for trouble; I just always needed to be busy.

This "alone time in Hawaii" was a true test of whether self-refection, meditation, and prayer were even possible for me now. Was I deluding myself by even signing up for this retreat?

It has always been my practice to carry a note pad with me and in this case I brought a fresh journal in anticipation of perhaps receiving divine guidance or inspiration to write during this journey. And that is exactly what I did. When I forgave myself for allowing my fears to almost overwhelm me, I began to realize I understood more than I gave myself credit for. Maybe I saw things that could help others passing through their own dark valley of loss. As inspiration emerged on the pages of my journal, so did the idea of writing this book. You might say it was born in the journal that I kept while I was there.

By the way, Elizabeth Gilbert's *Eat Pray Love* was also based on journals she kept while traveling through Italy, India, and Indonesia, although in her case the book wasn't exactly inspired *by* the journey. She imagined what the book would be before leaving on her journey and received a large advance from her publisher, which she used to finance the trip and write the book. Critics have questioned her work on that basis, but I believe there is inspiration in her pages. What I would say is that each of us must walk our own journey, but someone else's journey can help point the way. I hope my journey helps someone the way Ms. Gilbert's journey helped me.

So there I was on the Big Island, left to my own devices without distractions or interruptions. As the evening breeze cooled my skin, the thoughts and feelings began to flow. My mind raced back to many years earlier when I was widowed the first time. My therapist told me to keep a journal and to write down five things every day that I was grateful for. That was one of the best pieces of advice about working through the grieving process that I have ever received. It worked then and it worked now in Hawaii. My thoughts and feelings began to reshape themselves—more hopeful, expectant of good things rather than full of fear that my best times were over. I began to smile as I wrote.

I discovered that naming things to be grateful for is a good practice at any time, not just in times of extreme emotional distress. To be honest, most of us suffer emotional distress at many points in our lives, and it might not even be tied to any single event. It might just come on all of a sudden. When it does, remember to make your list of things to be grateful for; it will help lead you out of darkness.

Over the years from time to time I've continued that practice. It doesn't have to be new things every day. I have found over the years that although I've added new things to my lists, I have continued to be grateful for many of the same things.

I have continued to be grateful for my wonderful son, grandchildren, aunts and extended family. My girlfriends are invaluable in my life. And of course I am grateful for my good health and the ability to exercise and do something physical every day. After rehabbing from two major surgeries on my right leg within three years, I have a deep and imbedded appreciation for my ability to walk, swim, bicycle, do Qigong and yoga, play golf and live an independent life.

These are all things I took for granted until I realized I had almost lost them. These are all things that have continued to help me work through my healing journey. I say "work through" because I believe that we do have a choice as to how we want to proceed with our lives after a major change hits us—a change that we did not choose.

After suffering a loss or a major setback in life, we can pick up our marbles and go home. We can give up, which I believe we all do periodically and intermittently. But what is it that keeps bringing us back? What is it that gives us the motivation or the courage to continue when things get tough, when life goes off track?

FEELINGS OF WANTING TO GIVE UP . . .
IT'S A MORTAL SIN TO COMMIT SUICIDE

I still recall a few occasions when I couldn't chase away the thought of giving up on life and walking out into the depths of the dark blue ocean where the waves would carry me out to sea. It seemed like the answer or solution to the sadness and despair I was feeling. It would end my pain. But then I thought about the pain that I would be causing those that I left behind.

I was a hard working divorcee, raising a young child, struggling to make ends meet when this deep, desperate wave of depression first **swept** over me. My parents had invited me to join them to visit some friends of theirs at their beach condo back in the early 70s. As I was walking alone along the edge of the shore line, my thoughts were of escaping the pain.

Although I can't honestly recall the exact trials and tribulations that I was going through at that time, I knew that I was very depressed and felt unable to cope. Sometimes a series of smaller setbacks can drain our strength of spirit as surely as a large challenge like the loss of a loved one. So that evening I seriously considered allowing the waves to engulf me, to swim with the fish and the dolphins. Although I was a fairly strong swimmer and my parents would probably not have believed that it was an accident, I figured that a few gulps of salt water would sweep me out to sea. Obviously this was not a very rational thought process and probably would not have been a very peaceful or desirable way to leave this planet.

There were two things that held me back. Although my son was very young at the time and my parents adored him and would have raised him in my absence, I couldn't leave that stigma on him for the rest of his life. I have always believed that having my son saved my life. God does work in strange and interesting ways. He always seems to send us what we need, when we need it most. Alex is my only child and I don't know what I would have ever done, or would do, without him.

Since no one really knows what happens to us when we leave this world, I meditated on that a great deal, and still do for that matter. I was raised Catholic and was taught that it is a mortal sin to commit suicide. So if I did decide to check out early I would be doomed to eternal damnation in hell—whatever that is.

REINCARNATION

I had also studied and learned about reincarnation—not in the Catholic Church, of course. This is the belief that we have to keep coming back to a physical life on earth until we get it right. It is the belief that this life is not our first rodeo, which is why some people are more talented in certain areas then others. I believe that we all come into this life with certain talents and how we choose to use and develop our gifts is up to us.

We have been here before and done it before. Take Beethoven for example; he is the most obvious manifestation of someone who came into the life with an extraordinary talent and gift. There's no other explanation.

So, in other words we have to keep coming back until we get it right. I've always had this feeling or belief that if we leave this world miserable and unhappy we have to come back and deal with those feelings and issues in the next life.

I know it sounds crazy and there is no evidence or proof of this that I know of, but it is a theory that kept me from walking into the ocean many years ago—that and the stigma that it would have put on my son. Then there is the Catholic Church's teaching that suicide is a "mortal sin" punishable by eternal damnation. Intellectually, I didn't believe this, but as other Catholics have said, the church's ingrained teachings can be hard to overcome.

Life is about change and adjusting to the change ...

I guess I wasn't too far gone mentally if I could walk on the beach and do all of that rationalizing. Of course no one really, really knows the ultimate answers, but it's certainly something to think about. I've also studied and read about people who had near death experiences and their stories are compelling.

So why am I bringing up these deep rooted, depressing memories from years ago when I was divorced? Because I believe that the emotions and feeling that we experience when we lose our spouse through death or divorce can be very similar—even when we are the one who wants the divorce and believes that is necessary. I needed to remind myself of that. I have witnessed many friends recovering from both kinds of loss and I've seen that in either case the hurt was persistent and genuine.

In the months that followed my husband Tony's passing I walked the beach a lot and had those very same feelings and thoughts. I wanted to just walk out into the waves and allow them to engulf me. I thought about how long it would take before my lungs would fill and I would be overtaken.

Of course I didn't think about it for very long, or even very seriously. Because again, there was my son to consider and now I have grandchildren whom I adore and would never do that do. Then there is reincarnation and the "mortal sin" thing to think about. Yes, sometimes we can boost our spirits by recalling the things we are grateful for; at other times exploring the downside of our actions can help us right our ship.

As I said before, no one really knows, but I do believe that we are all here for a purpose, and until our creator decides that it is time for me to move on, I need to keep seeking my purpose and working on this great gift of life I've been given.

I've always felt that my purpose was to share information and make a difference in other people's lives, which is what motivated me to become an astrological coach, write my first book, this book, my monthly newsletters and my Facebook posts. What exhilarates me and keeps it all fresh is that my eyes open a little wider all the time as my understanding of the human condition continues to grow.

Life is about change and adjusting to the change and I have always found that astrology was a great tool to help me understand and work with the changes. I should say astrology and my belief in God. I believe that God created heaven and earth and all of the planets. I have learned and experienced that studying the movement of the planets as they affect all of us living on planet earth is a very helpful and important tool.

ASTROLOGY AND WRITING, MY WORKS OF LOVE . . .

In her book *Big Magic*, Elizabeth Gilbert wrote that whenever anyone tells her that they want to write a book in order to help others, she always thinks, "Oh please don't." She wrote that it was much better to write a book to entertain and help yourself.

She talks about the book she just happened to write based on her travel memoirs while trying to save herself after a failed marriage. Little did she know then that it would turn out to be a best seller and a very popular movie. I know her story certainly made an impression in my life. I can still remember when I read the book and couldn't wait to see the movie. Although I was in a good place in my life at the time—my husband had not been diagnosed yet—I still appreciated and could resonate with her story.

Everyone who hasn't been living on Mars or Venus knows it was called *Eat Pray Love*. I've seen it several times since the original release in the theater, and have found something new in it every single time.

So Elizabeth Gilbert's theory, which I totally agree with, is that if you do whatever it is that you love doing and it feeds your soul, it may end up, inadvertently, helping others. Elizabeth shared these words of wisdom from the theologian Paul Tillich, *"There is no love which does not become help."*

Ms. Gilbert also wrote, "If you can't do what you long to do, go do something else. Go walk the dog, go bake a peach cobbler, go paint some pebbles with brightly colored nail polish and put them in a pile. You might think it's procrastination, but—with the right intention—it isn't, it's motion. And any motion whatsoever beats inertia, because inspiration will always be drawn to motion. Do something. Do anything."

This got me thinking about how I have actually been doing this most of my life—looking for answers for myself that eventually became answers for others as well. I started studying astrology in the early 1980s at about the time when home computers became affordable and popular. If had not been for being able to calculate the astrological charts on a computer, I would never have pursued this career. It just made life so much easier. So as I pursued the career that was calling me, I found that the tools I needed to make it work seemed to appear. People talk about "being born at the wrong time," well I believe I was born at exactly the right time. Born in the right place at the right time—all of us have a better chance at living a joyful, fulfilled life if we believe that.

> When you reach for what you love doing, all good things are within your grasp

As I have become more and more evolved and

conscious of what I have learned and shared over the years, I feel very rewarded and deeply satisfied with my life's journey and my work.

The interesting thing is that Larry, my first late husband, was very supportive and encouraging about what I do. As a result my career evolved quickly. I was thriving in my work—reading for clients all over the country, teaching classes at the local college. There was a featured article about me in the local newspaper. I had found my niche and what fed my soul. I truly loved what I did and the people that I was blessed to work with.

A few years after Larry passed away I met Tony, who was very conservative. He really wasn't very keen on the idea of dating an "astrologer," which is probably why it took us five years to get married. Eventually I slowed down with my astrology work and he became more tolerant of what I did. But our life was busy, and my work took a back seat. Still, during this time I continued with my practice and when the time was ripe as Tony convalesced at home I wrote my first book, *An Astrologer's Journey*. And now in the aftermath of Tony's death comes the inspiration for my new book.

When you reach for what you love doing, all good things are within your grasp. Prevailing winds are always in your favor. That's what happened at the retreat in Hawaii; once I stopped resisting, the winds carried me exactly where I needed to go.

"It all works out in the end. If it isn't worked out, it isn't the end." — Traditional Wisdom

Chapter Six

SUN SIGNS AND PROCESSING LOSS
EACH IN THEIR OWN WAY AND TIME

It has been my observation and experience that we all heal—and hopefully grow and prosper—in different ways after experiencing a loss. The big question is, how can we make it an opportunity to go in a new and beautiful direction that we have never explored before. How do we learn to enjoy each sunrise again? How do we prosper in times of change, and especially after a loss.

Unfortunately, the longer we live the more loss and adjusting we have to deal with. But each loss can be a growing opportunity to bring out our strengths.

As a student and practicing professional astrologer for most of my adult life, I have found astrology it to be an invaluable tool. It has helped me to better understand myself and those around me, and to more effectively coach my clients.

Astrology is just another language in which to talk about our lives. Please forgive me, those of you who don't speak the language of "astrologese," But it's really just about timing and tendencies. Those who speak the language know what I mean. Those who don't, well, it's really quite simple, so follow along.

Each sun sign has its own personality, and so, accordingly, each individual has their own way of dealing with grief and loss. (Granted, the sign that the moon is in at the time of birth is also an important factor to consider, but I am going to keep it simple and focus on just the sun signs.)

This is what I have observed and experienced in working with my clients, friends and family members over these many years. The fire signs—Aries, Leo and Sagittarius—and air signs—Gemini, Libra, and Aquarius—tend to move forward at a quicker pace. It's not that they don't feel the sorrow and loss, they are just more open and tend to look for external distractions to help them through the process.

The water signs—Cancer, Scorpio and Pisces—have a tendency to withdraw, internalize and process their loss very personally. While the earth signs—Taurus, Virgo and Capricorn—tend to move in a slow organized direction. They will analyze and assess their financial situation to make sure they are secure.

Aries tend to have a pioneering, independent, competitive attitude. They especially like to move fast. They won't let any grass grow under their feet. If there is a way to fast forward the grieving and healing process they are all for. They are all about going full speed ahead. It doesn't mean that they don't feel the pain, they just have to keep moving while they are feeling it.

They feel better if they hit the ground running in the morning instead of lying in bed thinking about the past or feeling sorry for themselves. There's no time for self pity for an Aries. Some people may think they are insensitive or lacking in emotions, but the truth is they mask their pain with activity.

Since they are by their very nature a pioneering spirit, they are always up for starting and trying something new and different. This can be their salvation and greatest healing tool when dealing with a loss. I am not suggesting that they wake up the next morning after experiencing a loss as if nothing has even happened, but staying busy and having a plan of action is a terrific antidote for them.

Taurus natives tend to be patient, steadfast, and conservative. On the other hand, unlike Aries, they have a tendency to slowly process the change. They will first want to access their financial situation and stability. They are slower to deal with and accept changes in their life, especially the loss of a spouse—even when the handwriting is on the wall.

They find that working helps them to maintain stability, to stay grounded. They can find comfort in gardening and or just being in touch with nature. Those who were born with their sun or moon in the sign of Taurus usually find healing comfort when they have plants or flowers around them.

Fresh flowers can play an important role in the healing process for everyone, but especially for someone who has their sun or moon in Taurus. They may find comfort in food and may need to be careful about the extra pounds.

Geminis tend to be literary, versatile, adaptable, analytical and curious. This is another sign who likes to keep moving and get on with life. They find comfort and healing through connecting and interacting with their friends. Most Geminis are avid readers. They tend to be students of life. Reading about dealing with loss can be very healing for them. It is also helpful for them to journal, write, and share their experiences.

Cancers tend to be nurturing, receptive, cautious, reserved, and persevering. Family is everything for a Cancer. The loss of a family member, even an elderly grandparent or distant cousin, can be devastating for them. There is a tendency for them to hold their emotions inside with outbursts of tears of emotion. One of my Cancer friends said she invariably cries at weddings and funerals. Their deep sensitivity can affect their sleep pattern, their appetite, and their attention span. They find comfort in staying close to their home environment when grieving. Since they are initiators and activity oriented, home projects can be very healing for them.

Leos tend to be generous, ambitious, creative, entertaining, and optimistic. They need to let the child in them come out to play when they are dealing with a loss—let their creative juices flow. I can recall one Leo client who enjoyed painting, and after her husband passed away she painted the most beautiful landscapes. She even sold a few through a local studio.

Virgos tend to be ingenious, witty, studious, and methodical. They find comfort and stability in being organized and tending to the details of closure. A much older Virgo woman shared her story with a friend: when she lost her first child, a beautiful 18-month-old little boy, she was already pregnant with her second child. She was an excellent seamstress and began immediately making a layette for the child she was expecting. She said there were tears in every stitch. She also put away her little lost boy's clothes in her cedar chest, and never used them for another child, even though she ended up with four more children.

Libras tend to be persuasive, tactful, intriguing, social, charming, and can be indecisive at times. They usually find comfort and condolence with friends and social activities.

After wallowing in grief and generating their required tears, a Libra will get fed up and go do something that distracts, shifts, or redirects their energy. They cannot bear to feel like they have fallen into a well that they cannot climb out of. They do their best to create or manifest some balance. Social media can be a superb tool for creating and maintaining social, emotional, and healing connections, promoting the Libras' balance and healing over time.

Scorpios tend to be private, introspective, and very deep in their emotions. Although grief counseling could be very helpful for them, they may find it difficult to open up their emotions and let go. It's not easy for them to show or share their deep feelings, so it may take them a little longer to work through the healing process.

A friend of mine was dating a handsome, charming Scorpio man, but feared it would never work out because of his past. He had come home from his father's funeral to find another man in bed with his wife. They had a two-year-old little girl who meant everything to him. He had thrown his whole being into making a life for his young family. His reaction was to punch the intruder and file for divorce. He left a very good job and went on the road driving a truck for a major transport company. He took his little girl with him when school was not in session, and they listened to classical books on tape as he drove the highways. The daughter was now in college, and he had never re-married and never really gotten over the pain.

Sagittarius can be the eternal optimist and prefers to look at the glass half full rather than half empty. They are also the bachelor and bachelorettes of the zodiac. When experiencing a loss, a change of scenery can be just the ticket. They can enjoy traveling and being outdoors, especially if it is a trip to an exotic place they have never been before. Sagittarians are the philosophers of the zodiac, and can also be religious minded. A spiritual quest may be in order for some Sagittarians while they ponder life's lessons.

I have a Sagittarian friend who, after her husband left her, traveled to Egypt all alone from Florida to join up with a tour group of mostly Australians to cruise the Nile, explore the pyramids, and look for ancient symbols. She was overjoyed to find the Flower of Life in an ancient temple ruin, and came home feeling much better.

Capricorn — When down to brass tacks Capricorns can put their big boy pants on and become all business. Although they feel loss and the pain that comes with it, they tend to channel it in a productive, structured manner. There's no self pity party for a Capricorn. Granted, they have their moments where they break down in private, but for the most part they put up a pretty good front.

I can still recall when my father passed away after a very short lived lung cancer diagnosis. My mother, a Capricorn, worked with the help of a widow friend and family members to immerse herself in dismantling and preparing to sell their 30-foot motorhome. Capricorns tend to be great at organizing and delegating. Even when grieving, they can reorganize their life and make a plan of action.

My parents had traveled from Florida to Alaska, through Canada to Nova Scotia and all the states in between over a period of twenty years. They enjoyed a wonderful life together. But the task of dismantling their home on wheels was a monumental project which my mother embraced almost immediately. It gave her a focus and a purpose. Work and projects can be a great healing and growth avenue for Capricorns.

Work is a great antidote to help Capricorns through the healing and growth process. Like Aries, they do better when they are staying busy, although they do tend to be more organized than Aries.

Aquarius tend to be inventive, intellectual, diplomatic, and independent. They find comfort in social or humanitarian activities. They need to have a plan of action and set their goals. They enjoy their independence and like to do things their way. They can usually find a unique and different way to process their healing journey.

Pisces are intuitive, compassionate, introspective, loquacious, and clairvoyant. They have more of a tendency to want to withdrawal and escape. Sleeping is an excellent healing antidote for them. When a sweet Pisces lady lost her husband to a heart attack, she hardly got out of bed for a month. Then, a friend and silent business partner of her late husband offered her the opportunity to run the art gallery her husband had started. She threw herself into re-opening the gallery and spent the rest of her life fulfilling her late husband's dream.

Feeling sad is okay. It means you have great memories. You are remembering the good times and the fun you had together.

Chapter Seven

GETTING AMBUSHED AND CELINE DION

Again, just about the time you think you are healed and have all the tears and sadness behind you, something pops up that brings on another swale of tears. It doesn't have to be a major event. But for some reason holidays do seem to be a trigger.

It might not be a major holiday, like Christmas. It could be Memorial Day or 4th of July. As my neighbor said to me when I told her about my emotional setback on Memorial Day almost two years after Tony passed away, "Holidays are family times and when a family member is gone the void is most glaring on those days. Memorial Day weekend is when Tony and I would usually watch the French Open tennis tournament and the Indianapolis 500 on TV. I tried to watch the French Open alone, but it just wasn't the same without him.

My friend Joann who facilitates a bereavement

group at her church told me that feeling sad is okay. It means you have great memories. You're remembering the good times and the fun you had together.

MY HOUSEKEEPING IS A DIRECT REFLECTION OF MY EMOTIONAL STATE OF MIND

In addition to being great exercise, you can't cry when you're swimming. I have discovered that cleaning is also a good antidote and therapy for tears. I don't know why but there seems to be a calming and sense of satisfaction when I start vacuuming. I especially enjoy using my "Shark" steam cleaner on my tile floors. Now I know why I enjoy cleaning..

I recall watching an interview on TV years ago in which Celine Dion said that she enjoyed cleaning her own bathroom. She said she grew up dirt poor and this kept her humble and in balance. It was good therapy. She said it made her feel good. I thought that was kind of odd at the time, considering all of the fame and money she had. She could afford ten housekeepers, but she said it kept her life in perspective. This made me wonder how Celine Dion dealt with the death of her husband from cancer on January 14, 2016, only six months after Tony's passing. Then her brother, only 57 years old, died of the same kind of cancer two days later. I could picture the two of us seeking solace from our pain—me vacuuming and Celine on her knees cleaning her bathroom.

It seems that cancer has no financial boundaries. It doesn't care if you are wealthy and famous or poor as a church mouse.

Of course in the interest of research and the astrologer in me, I had to look at the dynamics of Celine Dion's horoscopes to appreciate and understand how she was handling and dealing with the sorrow of losing both her husband and brother within two days of each other. Where was she getting this inner strength and resolve?

Just to be clear, "a horoscope," as defined by Wikipedia, "is an astrological chart or diagram representing the positions of the Sun, Moon, planets, astrological aspects, and sensitive angles at the time of an event, such as the moment of a person's birth, for use by astrologers."

The very first thing I noticed is that Celine was born with her Sun in Aries conjunct Saturn. A conjunct means that the Sun and Saturn were traveling together in the sky at the time of her birth. This is an indication of a person who has self-restraint and great reserve. They typically will have strong discipline, personal strength, and persistence. They are controlled, hardworking, and determined. They are usually high achievers and usually have responsibility at a young age. Celine was one of 14 children.

With this in mind, I thought that she would hit the ground running despite the double loss and return to her career stronger than ever. Which is exactly what she did, at least for all outward appearance. We don't know about the tears she may have shed behind closed doors. I wasn't surprised to learn that after she gave herself a short time to grieve she began to live her new normal, going back on the road. Losing her husband of 21 years, René Angélil, to cancer in January, 2016 didn't come as a surprise, as he had been ill for some time; but as the Grammy-winning artist herself said: Her family lived with hope even when there was no hope.

She claimed to feel stronger after Rene's death,

perhaps because she believed he would always be with her.

Dion took a leave from her Las Vegas show in August 2014 to devote herself to caring for Angélil, who in addition to being the father of her three children had been her manager for the entirety of her storied career. And understandably, though it was valuable time spent together, watching his condition deteriorate was also a very painful experience.

> At first there was that feeling of maybe I could have done "this or that."

"I proved to Rene that he was there for me and I'm going to be there for him—and I'm still there for him," Celine said in her 2017 interview with Natalie Finn at eonline.com. "I took care of him the best way I could."

I personally feel and believe that knowing you did the very best that you could to care for your loved one is half the battle of moving forward. At first there was that feeling of maybe I could have done "this or that." Then come the thoughts of *if only* … I experienced those same thoughts and feelings when my mother passed away and both of my husbands. There was always something that I wish I would have said or done. And from what I have learned that's pretty normal.

The reality is that we all do the best we can. When our loved one is gone I don't believe they look back in judgment. I believe they are in a better space and a better place. This may sound a little cliché but if there is individual consciousness in the afterlife I have to believe it is a consciousness of pure love, not one of petty grievances—either imagined or real.

The first year after losing her husband, Celine said "love, faith, family and unsinkable strength" were her comfort. They had started out as a professional relationship—he served as Celine's manager—which later turned romantic leading to a lavish wedding in 1994.

As Celine continues to get used to her new normal, the Grammy winner is revealing some of the final words she shared with her husband. "When he passed, I stood by his side and I said, 'You know what, it's okay, you know you didn't deserve to suffer that much.' He was cold. I said, 'It's enough, it's enough of suffering. You gave so much, you don't deserve that,'" she explained. "I said, 'I'm fine, the kids are fine, okay, everything is going to be okay. You taught me, you taught me well. I'm going to use it.' And that's what I do every day—so Rene will never die."

Although we are not all Grammy winners, I believe we can appreciate and be inspired by Celine Dion when she made an emotional return to the stage in Las Vegas, just over a month after her husband René died while battling throat cancer. In addition to her husband's death, Dion's brother, Daniel Dion, died two days after Angélil.

The singer honored her late husband of over 20 years with a moving montage of photos and video that can be seen on her website, celinedion.com. As reported by Carly Ledbetter of Huffpost, the tribute also included an emotional message. "I understood that my career was in a way his masterpiece, his song, his symphony," said the text in the tribute. "The idea of leaving it unfinished would have hurt him terribly. I realized that if he ever left us, I would have to continue without him, for him."

The singer teared up a few times during that first night back on stage and broke down during her signature song "All by Myself." She finished the night in true professional fashion with the crowd totally on her side.

I HAVE ALWAYS ADMIRED AND FELT A STRONG CONNECTION WITH CELINE DION

I guess I should mention why I especially found her horoscope to be interesting and motivational. I am also an Aries but instead of Saturn in conjunction to my Sun, it is on my ascendant, which has a very similar astrological interpretation as Saturn conjunct the Sun. And of course, I admired the way she bounced back from her loss so quickly while still honoring the memory of her lost loved ones.

Although I wasn't doing a concert in Las Vegas a month after Tony passed away I also hit the ground running with my professional astrological and volunteer work. I didn't hide. I held onto my memories of him—of us—as precious jewels and opened myself to what would come next in life. Yes, there were times like that first Memorial Day weekend when the memories were sharp and even painful. And because I continued the social life I had with my girlfriends, I took the chance that some unintentional comment would trigger a burst of sadness. But this is life—full of beautiful possibilities but not without its risks.

Be diligent in your practice. Whatever it may be—Qigong, Tai chi, Yoga, Meditation or some other form—do it several times a week.

Chapter Eight

THE IMPORTANCE OF A SPIRITUAL PRACTICE

As I described in an earlier chapter it was a week-long Qigong retreat in Hawaii that was my turning point toward recovery, or rebirth—however you want to see it.

It all began in April of 2016 when my dear friend Krista, with whom I have a Jupiter connection, invited me to a weekend Qigong Healing Forum presented by Jeff Primack in Daytona Beach in April of the year following Tony's passing. That weekend began a transformation for me that truly blossomed in Hawaii a little later. When you have a Jupiter connection with someone, as I do with Krista, it is like that person is a guardian angel for you. They seem to always be there for you when you need them most, and they are an inspiration. Be ready to accept such gifts that often arrive though friends. I will always appreciate them and never regret that I did.

Many of us have those kinds of weekend experiences at seminars or retreats that may last no more than two or three days, up to a week. The question is how to take that elevated feeling you leave with and make it real every day of your life. How do you make it last? The answer, I believe, is you need to have a practice whatever it may be. It could be Qigong, Tai chi, yoga, one of the many forms of meditation, or even prayer. Do it daily or at least several times a week. It may not blow your socks off like a week in Hawaii, but the cumulative effect will be greater for bringing joy and peace of mind into your life.

So after doing some research about Qigong my interest was piqued enough to register for the weekend forum. I learned that, *Qigong is a lifestyle that harnesses energy from special movements, breathing methods and uses specific foods to reverse specific diseases. Everyone has a healing hand and anyone can benefit with practice.*

I came across this quote from Dr. Rick Agel MD and AP Surgeon of Atlanta, Georgia, "This system combines Qigong with Breathing Exercises that are *phenomenally energetic.* In thirty years of practicing Tai Chi, this is the strongest chi I've ever felt."

So I went to the weekend forum, full of anticipation, but not knowing exactly what to expect. Believe me when I say that I was not disappointed.

It was exactly what I needed. I was introduced into a whole new world of personal empowerment. The first night of the conference I received my first "gift," the "nine step breathing technique," which was an amazing relaxation tool.

It seems that most of us just "breathe." Or we think we are breathing, but are we really taking deeply inhaled breaths into our abdomen? It is amazing what nine deep breath inhalations will do for our mind and body.

It's not complicated. We simply sat in a chair and took a deep breath as we were sitting up straight and leaned forward as we exhaled. We did this nine times at a fairly quick pace. Try it. Remember to sit up straight in a meditative position—back straight and shoulders relaxed—as you inhale, then lean forward as you exhale, and return to upright for the next inhale. It does tend to make you a little light headed so you have to be careful before you stand up.

We also learned about and experienced the benefits of the power breathing, which brought out emotions so deep that I didn't even know they were there. As we were lying flat on our mats on the floor, we took in a very deep breath and then lifted up on our elbows to exhale quickly. We did this 50 times under Jeff's count and direction. This was another amazingly powerful exercise. Again, you had to be careful before standing as it made you feel very light headed.

It was about feeding every part of my being.

I have been practicing yoga and meditating for years. I went through the Transcendental Meditation course when I was going through my divorce in the 70s. I thought I was an experienced and seasoned meditator, but I had never experienced the serene feeling that Qigong gave me. It was even better than a couple glasses of wine or a martini. I would come home at night after a full day and evening of practicing and absorbing this new discipline, feeling a sense of a euphoric high.

I did not need or want to turn on the TV or even listen to music. I experienced a feeling of serenity and introspection. I was truly in touch with my healing journey. I was in a good place.

Once again Krista, my *guardian*, had come to my rescue when she introduced me to this practice.

The weekend was not only about physical and mental exercise it was about nutrition and healthy eating. It was about feeding the mind, body and spirit, which as it turned out was exactly what I needed to help me along my healing journey at time in my life.

People use the word "holistic" quite freely, but when one really practices with a thought to all parts of your being—mind, body and spirit—it brings a peace through internal unity that can't be reached when one part of the equation is missing.

I learned about the benefits of eating red pepper paste, which is very high in antitoxins, cardiovascular, and anti-aging benefits and happens to be delicious. I use it like mayonnaise or an appetizer dip. Although it takes a little while to make, I found the process to be very therapeutic and enjoyable. I even started making extra to share with my neighbor who also enjoys it (*see recipe on Page 182*).

The other thing I really found beneficial was the "Anti-Inflammation Smoothie," which consists of cherries, cucumber, papaya, ginger root and pineapple. In addition to being delicious, I found that it really helped my arthritis (*see receipt on page 40*).

All of this happened at the weekend retreat in Daytona Beach, so as you can guess, I was inclined to sign up for the week in Hawaii. But I wanted more information and confirmation about my decision to make this leap into a new world and new experience across the Pacific Ocean, so I went home and quickly ran my astrology chart for the dates of the retreat.

An astrology chart would show me were all the plants would be at the time of the retreat and I could compare it to what was going on in my birth chart, so I could get a better appreciation and understanding of the timing and if this was a favorable time to do this.

I couldn't have been more excited about what I saw, although not really surprised. I am always amazed at how when we take one brave step forward the universe takes our hand and walks with us. As Julia Cameron, author of *the Artist's Way*, likes to say, "Leap and the net will appear."

After all, I knew what an amazing impact the conference in Daytona Beach had on my life, so I could only imagine what a week at a retreat in Hawaii would have on my life.

After my husband passed away I continued working with my astrology clients and helping other people with the challenges in their life. I continued teaching and scheduling workshops. I continued to stay busy and keep my mind occupied.

Since I was still healing and adjusting to the loss of my husband, I felt I needed this opportunity, this retreat, to work on myself and regain my inner peace and strength. I say *regain*, which I think most people who've suffered loss hope for. The surprise waiting was for me was that I was destined not only to regain my former self, but to surpass the person I was before.

"Don't cry because it's over, smile because it happened." — Dr. Seuss

Chapter Nine

RECONNECTING AND REMEMBERING

It has been and is my feeling that there is a great deal of comfort and satisfaction in reconnecting and revisiting.

In my former life, many years ago before I met Tony, I was director of sales and marketing at a resort in Stuart, Florida.

It was during this cycle in my life that I took a Transcendental Meditation (TM) class and began the practice of daily meditation. I was introduced to the work of Edgar Cayce, one of the most prolific psychics in the twentieth century. I studied Tarot Cards, dream analysis, and numerology in addition to continuing my astrological studies. I was a true seeker, and in many ways I still am. There's always something new to discover.

And then came an exciting breakthrough. I met a woman named Betty Riley who helped change my life. She was a psychic medium who had written a book called *A Vale Too Thin – Out of Control.* Her true experience of reincarnation is one of the best documented cases on record. Without going too deeply into Betty Riley's story, she was a psychic of remarkable ability whose awareness of past lives manifested in her present life.

I know many people find such phenomena hard to believe, but those people have not met Betty Riley. Her ability to see things far beyond the limitations of most people was so powerfully real that university researchers sought to find a viable explanation.

So when Betty saw something in me that I had not seen in myself, and encouraged me to pursue my astrological gifts, I knew that my path had been chosen.

And, as I envisioned taking my life's work to a higher level, I also understood that the thing which made it a higher level was the opportunity for helping and working with others.

I continued to thrive with my love of helping others through astrology. My studies and practice continued to grow. Then I met Tony. As wonderful as he was, he had reservations about me being an astrologer, which is why we dated for five years before we got married. Eventually he began to learn and understand more about what I was doing. He understood that there was not a conflict between God, religion and astrology. So we were able to live happily ever after until …

Of course, given the central role she had played in my life, I reconnected and reached out to Betty Riley after Tony passed. She lived in Atlanta and I lived in Florida, so we were only able to talk on the phone, which I found to be very comforting.

Almost Two Years Later

Although we had always kept in touch through email and phone calls, I hadn't seen Betty in over 20 years. When she told me she was going to do her "swan song" in Milwaukee, I immediately said "I'll be there!" I had previously done an astrology program for the Edgar Casey group in Milwaukee, which is where she would be speaking.

I loved the group and knew that reconnecting face to face with Betty after all of these years was going be invaluable and instrumental in my healing journey. It was everything I hoped it would be. I scheduled a reading with her which was very enlightening and helpful.

I found it very interesting that it directly correlated with the information that I was seeing in my astrology chart. She didn't tell me anything that was foreign or uncomfortable to me. One of the things that she told me that struck a chord with me was that I should write another book. She actually validated that I was on the right track and path with my healing journey.

I believe we all need validation in our life no matter how strong or confident we are. And we should all have our "go to" people. Our "go to" people can be different people at different times in our life. And quite often they get as much from giving to us as we receive from them.

As I have said before, I believe everyone is in our life for a reason, even if it is only a season. Thank you, Betty Riley for being in my life. My "go to" person was a mentor in the field which I made my life's career. Yours might be someone different according to your beliefs—maybe a pastor, or former professor—someone you respect who isn't necessarily a close personal friend.

During Betty's workshop she mentioned that when she lived in Florida many years ago, she would always walk on the beach when she was searching for answers or looking for comfort. She said she believes in God and, "when I look at the magnitude of the ocean my problems seemed so small." Her belief in God is what got her thought the tough times.

She also believes in the importance of meditation and makes it a practice to meditate daily. When you pray, you talk to God, but when you meditate, you listen to God.

She said it's important to let the ego go when meditating. Shut everything down. Just allow the mind to be quiet and listen. Granted this does take practice, but it does develop with time and patience. Some people find it easier to meditate when they are walking. They say walking quiets their mind. Betty says just do whatever works best for you.

> **Don't let someone else's beliefs limit you—whether it is an individual, an institution, or the culture.**

One of the books that Betty Riley referred to during her presentation in Milwaukee was Ruth Montgomery's *How to Communicate with Spirit.* Ruth Montgomery was a journalist with a long career as a reporter and syndicated columnist in Washington, DC.

Later in life she became a celebrated psychic and author of numerous books on spiritual subjects. During the 1960s and '70s Montgomery became a regular on the morning talk show circuit, and was for a time a household name. She was a pioneer that helped make Betty Riley's career possible.

One of the things I have learned from my studies is that if you can imagine it, you can reach it. Don't let someone else's beliefs limit you—whether it is an individual, an institution, or the culture. The most rewarding path is always the one you choose for yourself.

What motivates us to do what we do? For me it is the desire to stay mentally and physically healthy and stay independent.

Chapter Ten

EXERCISE: THE MULTI-PURPOSE THERAPY

Exercise and physical activities have always played a major role in my life. Sometimes it plays a more prominent role than other times, but it's always been at the top of my list of thing to make time for. So when going through stressful or distressful times I kick it into high gear.

When my husband Larry passed away in 1993, I started training for mini triathlons with my son. It just so happened that Mars, the energizer bunny was dancing with my Jupiter, the guardian angel and expander, opposing my Sun. So I was I was charged and highly motivated.

I believe it was a saving grace for me. It helped me to move forward physically and emotionally. People will say that it's "good to stay busy and take your mind off it," but it's more than that. There's something about movement of the muscles, especially the large muscles, that has its own magic. It gets the endorphins and adrenalin going. It can be euphoric and mentally healing. At least I have always found it be.

Then in 2015 when Tony passed away, Mars, was in conjunct with Uranus in my astrological chart. For those who speak the language, you know that this can be very conducive for strong bursts of energy. So guess what. I decided to join a second gym. I had been a member of the YMCA for years because they had an Olympic pool which I loved. I felt that I was ready to step up my workout with additional activities that the other gym offered. And besides, moving into a new environment felt very appealing.

I knew that triathlons were no longer in my future, due to some physical limitations, but I could still swim, spin, do yoga, and ride my bike on the beach.

During those days of recovery in the first year after, swimming attracted me more than any of the others. After all, it was impossible to cry while I was swimming, so I swam a lot. And since swimming is one of the best exercises you can do for your body, I was loving it. There's no stress on your body when you're in the water.

Swimming seems to always be there as the perfect exercise. It was the very first thing that I could get back to doing when I was recovering from hip replacement and quadriceps surgeries. Of course I didn't have these surgeries at the same time.

I could actually swim before I could walk after I had my quadriceps reattached to my knee bone. That was fun. Fortunately, Tony was still with me during that time. Although he was not Nancy nurse, he did the best he could, which was to call my aunt and uncle in California to come stay with us.

Fortunately, I was a fast healer and bounced back quickly from my surgeries. I expected, or at the very least, hoped to bounce back emotionally after my husband passed away. But broken hearts seem to take longer to mend then hips and knees do. I know that now.

Extra "bennies" from staying fit and working out

What motivates us to do what we do? For me it is the desire to stay mentally and physically healthy—the desire to maintain my independence until I am at least 101 so that my son and/or grandchildren do not need to take care of me.

It's the desire to stay healthy so that I can live and work as much as possible with compassion for others. Helping is why I chose my profession and why I write. I recommend it as a motivation in life. Of course, you never know when your opportunity will come to influence someone in a small but positive way.

So yes, working out was fun for me and when it brought me a little notoriety in my home town I had to smile. The Community Editor from our local paper interviewed me for a special interest feature about "working out and staying young." I share it here with you in hopes of expressing my desire to see just one more person start on a path to fitness.

Work out, stay young: That's the Kelly Lowe way

Emily Blackwood, Community Editor for the Ormond Beach Observer

Every day, Kelly Lowe has a different plan. On Monday and Wednesday she swims for 45 minutes. She rides the stationary bike at Gold's Gym Tuesday and Thursday and then takes a yoga class.

And on Friday, she plays golf. "I do something active every day," she said. "And golf definitely counts."

During the weekend, the Ormond Beach resident keeps up her routine with something a little more low key, like a walk on the beach. It is the weekend after all.

"I've always tried to stay physically active," Lowe-Pirkle said with a smile. "Varying exercise makes sure my body doesn't get overworked."

For those who are just starting out, the lifelong astrologist and published author says to start off with doing one activity that you like just two days a week. Rather than form this big fitness plan, make small goals that you know you can easily attain. That will keep you motivated to do more.

When it comes to eating healthy, Lowe-Pirkle advocates for staying away from sugars. She advises to eat low-carb foods.

"I try to stay away from sugar," she said. "Not that I don't have wine, but wine doesn't count."

Her diet consist of a lot of veggies, fruits and proteins. She says salmon and celery are some of the best things you could eat.

While the motivation to stay consistent with

a healthy lifestyle can sometimes be hard to maintain, Lowe-Pirkle said she does so because it keeps her feeling young and energetic.

"You're going to be able to think better," she said. "Your attitude is going to be better. It's your state of mind that is so rewarding."

I must say that this article certainly gave me an added boost and inspired me to continue my regimen, which has served me well. My commitment to exercise has not only helped me to move forward emotionally it has helped me to stay strong, fit and healthy.

Put your faith in knowing that whatever your pain, the sun will rise in the morning.

You don't have to be a triathlete or even join a gym. Any regular form of exercise can be mentally and physically healing and helpful. Even a walk around the block can lift your spirits and help your attitude. Ask yourself, "What is the one thing I can do right now, given who I am and the resources I have?" Do that one thing, then go a step further from there.

A SOURCE OF ENERGY TO LIFT BODY, MIND AND SPIRIT

Another case in point that comes to mind is a gentleman I met after his wife of many years passed away. He shared with me that he had put on a lot of extra pounds while he was caring for her during her extended illness. His cholesterol was high. His blood pressure was high, and he got absolutely no exercise. His diet was, to put it simply, atrocious. He was on a fast track for disaster. Then he became motivated and interested in swimming laps in the pool.

Five laps a day was all he could handle the first week.

After a few months he was up to twenty laps. He could see and feel the excess pounds melting away just by changing his diet and incorporating swimming into his daily routine. Not only did he look better, he said he felt so much better. He was healthier. He had more energy. His anxiety and depression started to subside. He was beginning to feel and look like a new person. In fact, he was a new person. He dropped three sizes in his pants and went from an extra-large to medium shirt size.

Then he decided to join the gym and work out on the treadmill and weight machines. He even joined a Yoga class. He was embracing his new self. He loved this new source of energy that seemed to feed his body and mind and lift his spirits. As his exercise regimen increased, his oxygen flow also seemed to increase. He was on a roll and he loved it. The last time I spoke with him he had lost over 50 lbs. He said he felt great and was enjoying the compliments. He was physically and mentally a new and different person. More importantly, he was, once again, a person he liked and enjoyed being.

Exercise can be a wonderful tool, good for so many things including renewing your enthusiasm for life. It can certainly help us enjoy the sunrises during a morning walk—if you can get up early. Put your faith in knowing that whatever your pain, the sun will rise in the morning and you will be given the blessing of another day.

"I think it's true what they say: Life really is a journey—and it's not always easy to know which maps to trust, or what to pack for the trip. But whatever the weather, wherever the road leads, I think the best possible traveling advice would be this: Bring a friend." — Keely Chace

Chapter Eleven

GIRLFRIENDS ARE FOREVER

As I reflect on where I have been on my path and consider how I have connected with so many fellow travelers on my healing journey, I am in constant amazement and appreciation of the dynamic effect that girlfriends can have on helping us through this process. I don't know what I would have done—or would do now—without them.

The loving support and connection with family is certainly very important, but as we get older most of our children take on a life and responsibility for their own family, spouses, children, and careers. They haven't stopped loving you, but they are at a different time of life, busy maintaining and running their own households. To put it simply, they are writing their own family narrative in which you are an important character, but not the lead role.

I have known people who never had children for whom friends become more like family than many families. Girlfriends often seem to form an exceptional bond, especially after they lose their spouse. Maybe that's why widows don't seem to feel the desire or need to remarry as quickly as widowers do . . . or do they?

You may have heard the saying "widows mourn, men replace." It sounds like common sense. If it is true, no one had actually proved it so, or explored why it might be that way.

We're all aware of the demographic imbalance between men and women, but is there more to it? I found a fascinating article called *The Desire to Date and Remarry Among Older Widows and Widowers* by Deborah Carr at Rutgers University that specifically tries to answer three questions about later life match-ups: (a) Do widowed men and women differ in their preferences for dating and remarriage in the short term (6 months) and longer term (18 months) following spousal loss? (b) To what extent can the observed gender gap in re-partnering be explained by gender differences in the perceived benefits and strains of romantic relationships, compared to other forms of social support? *and* (c) Is the fulfilled (or unmet) desire for a romantic relationship associated with psychological adjustment to spousal loss?

The entire research-based article, which is easy to read, can be found at *http://www.rci.rutgers.edu/~carrds/publications/remarriage.pdf*

In some ways the article can only tell us what the numbers say about how people behave after loss, what is the most common outcome. But "the numbers" don't have to predict what happens to you. It is my belief and experience that we can design our own outcome. One thing you can count on is if you don't design your life yourself, someone else—or circumstances—will design it for you. That sounds a little scary.

I'm not saying you should picture yourself as a lone wolf bravely crossing the horizon on a high ridge. No, we all need companions—co-conspirators if you will. I have been very fortunate in that I consider myself to be a very healthy and independent person, but there was an occasion a couple of years after my husband passed away that I found myself in an emergency situation when I developed a pinched nerve in my upper back. This is probably the most excruciatingly painful experience that I had ever experienced, next to shearing my quadriceps tendon a few years before my Tony passed away.

> I keep my eye focused on who is here now, not on who is missed but gone.

The difference with the sheared tendon was that Tony was with me. I never felt alone. I was in a great deal of pain, but I wasn't alone. And that was important to me.

When I made the trips to the emergency room with the pinched nerve drama, I was fortunate and blessed to have my girlfriends' support. It was as if the universe saw I was in need and knew just who to send to help me. Another of my girlfriends with whom I have a Jupiter connection, once again came through for me spending five hours in the ER with me.

I can still recall years ago while I was married to Larry, who was suffering more and more from congestive heart failure. I could see the handwriting on the wall but didn't have the kind of close girlfriends I could turn to. Perhaps it was a life habit from my youth. Growing up as a military brat, we moved every two years, so I never really developed lifelong girlfriends. It was during this time in my life, as Larry's health slipped away, that I decided to join Beta Sigma Phi, a professional sorority.

As my husband was going in and out of the hospital I felt a strong need for bonding with girlfriends. I didn't let that feeling pass without acting on it. And I can say now that decision to act set off a chain of events that ended with some wonderful lifelong girlfriends. I don't think I could have survived without their love and support over the years. Of course my parents were always there for me, but they too have passed on.

What I keep my eye focused on now is not who is missed and gone, but rather who is here. I do appreciate the friendship and support of my girlfriends.

AND THEN YOU MEET SOMEONE . . .
IF YOU'RE HUNGRY, HERE'S FOOD FOR THOUGHT

After months or years of "being alone" and enjoying your time with your "girlfriends" you meet someone special. He fits your intention list. He's the answer to your prayers and dreams. So what happens to the connection that you had with your girlfriends? This has the potential to get a little sticky, I feel that I'd be remiss in not addressing this issue.

One example that comes to mind is a friend who fell off the face of the earth when, after five years of being a widow, met the man of her dreams. Although I was very happy for her, I missed our connection and friendship. As great as her marriage might have been, wouldn't she have been even richer if she continued to nurture the love and friendship of girlfriends?

Life certainly does change when you meet someone, but what happens if it doesn't work out and you've kicked all your girlfriends to the curb. I guess that's why I feel it is important to keep a balance in your life even when you think you have met Mr. Wonderful.

Girlfriends are forever and, well, men seem to come and go—for whatever reason, no matter how long they stay. At least that has been my experience. So don't lose touch with your girlfriends no matter how wonderful "he" is.

> *"A man does what he can; a woman does what a man cannot."*
>
> — Isabel Allende, *Inés of My Soul*

Chapter Twelve

MEN ARE FROM MARS, WOMEN ARE FROM VENUS OR IS IT THE OTHER WAY AROUND

I don't believe in accidental or chance meetings. I believe that timing is everything and when people come into our lives—even if it is for a few minutes or an hour—there is a message or a reason.

A few years after Tony passed away I was having my routine oil change on my car, which I discovered was long overdue. I was normally very good about staying on top of this, but somehow it just got away from me this time. I am very fortunate to have a long time trusted mechanic who has taken care of Tony and me for many years.

He and his wife, Debbie, run a "two man show" repair shop. Patrick runs the back of the house, the garage, and Debbie runs the front of the house, the office. I don't know what I would have done or would do without them. I believe that every widow needs a good, reliable mechanic. There's nothing worse than feeling like you're being taken advantage of but you can't prove it one way or the other. You don't know what's wrong with your vehicle but you do know it has to be fixed. Trust is everything and it is so comforting to have a first class, top notch trusted mechanic when you are left alone—someone who is not going to rip you off or take advantage of you.

In addition to routine maintenance on my car I know that Patrick always has my back in an emergency. He's almost like a family friend I can rely on. Like when I accidently cut a corner too close in my car, ran over a gutter and blew out my tire, he was the first person I called. Fortunately I was able to crawl at low speed to his shop. He doesn't have a tow truck and I was too impatient to wait for AAA.

Back to my long overdue routine oil change . . . I left my car with Patrick and was walking into their little waiting room when a man who I thought was also dropping off his car walked in behind me. I thought this a little odd because Debbie never scheduled two appointments at the same time.

I sat down and immediately pulled out my cell phone to check my messages and social media. While I was looking down at the phone, the man struck up a conversation and said he had forgotten his cell phone at home. I'm thinking he probably doesn't have a wife or she would have reminded him to take it. I know Tony never seemed to remember on his own to take his cell phone when he was going out. I hated it when I'd try to call him and the phone was sitting on the dining room table, so I'd make it a point to always remind him to take it.

The man seemed like he wanted to talk to me, so I put my phone away. There was nothing that couldn't wait. As it turned out, he was not having his car serviced. He was waiting for someone else who was dropping off their car so he could give them a ride.

The person dropping off their car never materialized and an hour later we were still talking. I learned that his wife passed away a little over a year earlier and he was having a really hard time with it. It still almost brought tears to his eyes to talk about her. They had been married for over forty years. She had dementia and Parkinson's, so he took care of her for several years before she passed. Those final years had been completely absorbing for him. It was easy for me to identify with him.

I could see that he was still struggling and having a very difficult time adjusting. It has been my observation that men typically do have a much more difficult time dealing with life without their spouse, perhaps because they are often the ones accustomed to being taken care of for the most part. I realize that there are exceptions, but women are usually the ones who run the household—especially the kitchen.

So I immediately put on my counseling hat and asked him what he had been doing since she passed. He said "nothing, not a darn thing." We talked and talked and talked for over an hour. I mostly asked questions and listened. He even laughed a few times which he said he hadn't done in a long time.

I shared with him that I was an astrological counselor and asked him for his birthday, which he was happy to share. I even offered to give him a copy of my first book, *An Astrologer's Journey*, which he enthusiastically accepted. When I realized that he was a Cancer sun sign, I could certainly empathize with him and feel his pain. Cancers are usually very focused on their home and family life. They are nurturers and comfort creatures. They enjoy being home and sharing their life with someone. I could appreciate and understand how devastated this gentleman was. Without his wife, life felt distorted to him. I could see how much he was still suffering. But I felt that our "chance" meeting was very helpful for him. I could see his face soften and his eyes light up as were talking.

As it turned out, there had been a miscommunication about the meeting location with the person who he was to give a ride from the repair shop. I learned later that the person he was waiting for in the wrong place at the wrong time was his pastor at church. So for over an hour this struggling survivor was in the wrong place getting just what he needed—a sympathetic and knowing ear. It was an hour I believed to be very well spent for both of us. He was a widower who was still going through a very rough time and needed someone to talk with, and I had been down that road and was farther along in my healing process. I felt that he was lifted up and encouraged by our "chance" meeting and conversation.

It was really no surprise to me when I went home and calculated his astrology chart and discovered that we had several very supportive and favorable astrological planetary connections. For those who speak the language, we had a Mars/Sun and Pluto/Venus connection. Although we were like two ships who happen to be passing in the in the middle of the ocean, I believe our paths were destined to cross so that I could perhaps help him during his healing journey. The central theme of the story he shared with me was that his wife had been sick for a very long time and his life had been devoted to takin care of her. Her care was his purpose for living and with her gone now he felt lost. He was taking anti-depressants and trying to put his life back together again but was yet to discover a new purpose.

So he wasn't supposed to there, but he was. I was two months overdue in getting my routine oil change, or I wouldn't have been there either. As I said, I don't believe in coincidence. We did become phone friends, and I'd like to think I was able to contribute some helpful, healing conversation for him.

EVERYONE TRAVELS THEIR OWN JOURNEY
AND HEALS IN THEIR OWN TIME.

Men react differently to loss in a variety of ways. One of those ways is how long they wait before seeking someone new. Simply put, most men don't stay on the market very long.

Of course this is a generalization, but I have noticed that men are more inclined to find a companion much sooner than women do after losing their spouse. Maybe it's because at a certain age there are more women who are available then men. Statistics show that men die first. Maybe it's because women are more likely to marry older men. I know I always did. Availability of women in various age groups increases the size of the pool.

But then there are exceptions, like my mother. My father was three years younger than her. She never forgave him for getting lung cancer and leaving her. She never in a million years thought that he would die first, which is probably why she never got over it. Even though she was a strong women, she eventually gave up.

On another note, one of the men I interviewed whose wife of forty-five years had passed away six months earlier, shared with me that a Jewish women who lived in his building was a *Yenta,* which anyone familiar with *Fiddler on the Roof* knows is a Jewish/Yiddish word for a woman who is a matchmaker. She had a list of women who she wanted him to meet. Little did she know that he had already met someone who he was interested in.

Everyone, it seems, has a friend they want a widower to meet.

Although he was deeply shaken and saddened by the loss of his wife, who had been sick for many years prior to her passing, he was motivated to move forward with his life in the present—without waiting out some arbitrary time on the sidelines. He took specific steps to get there, including attending bereavement classes at his church. He believes the classes helped give him a context for understanding what he was feeling.

He shared with me that he was in a pretty bad place for the first couple of months, but his faith and a conviction that she was in a much better place and no longer suffering helped him through the dark days.

The gentleman's story of how he found someone new before the *yenta* could make her first move sort of reminded me of the Jimmy Buffett song "Everyone's Got a Cousin in Miami." Everyone, it seems, has a friend they want a widower to meet—especially if the man is financially secure and enjoys taking a woman out to dinner, dancing, and sending flowers—as this man did. I knew that he certainly wouldn't stay on the market very long. But unfortunately he jumped into a relationship too quickly after losing his wife and was blindsided by the consequences. He was not as compatible with his new love interest as he thought he would be. So, he then had to deal with recovery from what he called a "failed relationship" within the same year of losing his wife.

It just seems to me that there are a lot more people eager to be matchmakers for men than there are for women. But then, I have to remind myself that I met both of my late husbands through friends. One never really knows where opportunities may appear if that is what you are looking for. Or you may decide that you just enjoy your own space and your own company.

It pays to keep an open mind and an open heart. Often when a couple looks back on the winding paths they followed to find each other they can't help but say "it was meant to be."

In one way, however, men and women are alike after the loss of a spouse. It has been my observation, and research shows, that for both men and women those who have been in a happy marriage or relationship choose not to remain alone after their partner is gone. There is something very special for them about having a deep connection with another person. But then it is okay if you do not choose to go down that path.

Give yourself permission to be yourself—or by yourself if that feeds your soul.

I'm not advocating that everyone start dating right away. There is a lot to be said for allowing time to grieve. The timing is different for everyone. It takes as long as it takes, but often times meeting someone special who understands and appreciates where you are coming from can make the healing journey a little more palatable even if it only temporary.

"You're not a virgin and you didn't get divorced, but suddenly there's this thing you can start doing again with someone who is not your husband." – Ann Benjamin, *Life After Joe*

Chapter Thirteen

SEX, DRUGS AND ROCK AND ROLL

Sex is a great distraction if that's what you are looking for.

Several women shared with me that getting involved in an intense romance served as a perfect antidote or smoke screen during the grieving process after they lost their husband (or after a divorce, which could be another book in of itself).

Well maybe it wasn't quite perfect—more of a Band-Aid to cover their wounds than genuine healing. But it certainly was an effective distraction even if it turned out to be a painful roller-coaster ride. The highs were very high and lows were very low, as my friend Zoe described it to me.

Zoe found comfort after he husband's death with a man she had known for several years who was a family friend. Although there was a mutual attraction, there was never anything physical between them. After all, he was married and so was she. And she was very much in love with her husband. She said that before her husband's death she never even imagined them being any more than just friends.

Then about six months after her husband passed, she was going through grief counseling and was well on her way to what she thought and felt was her successful healing journey when she ran into him. It was like a bolt of lightning hit her. Was he to be her savior, her port in the storm? Would he be a devastating distraction she might regret later, or perhaps a catalyst to help her through her grieving process?

Maybe he was to be all of these. After all, they had known each other for years, so it wasn't like she was having an affair with a stranger. There was comfort in that. She felt safe and fulfilled when they were together. The sex was exciting and it made her feel alive again. It had been a very long time since she enjoyed the soothing intimacy that she felt with him. Her husband had been sick for several years and she had forgotten what it was like to experience passion and physical satisfaction with a man.

Oh, did I mention that he was still married. Not happily, but legally nonetheless. He was probably, maybe, going to get a divorce some day after he got his business affairs in order and his children were grown. But in the meantime, none of that mattered to her. This euphoric feeling she was experiencing was so much better than the pain and agony she had been feeling after her husband passed away.

Zoe realized that she was in a transitional state on her healing journey, and he was a welcome distraction. She wasn't looking for a husband, and a good lover seemed to satisfy her needs and fill the void in her life—the void in her heart and her body.

But then, as often happens in a situation like this, the reality set in that her affair was only a distraction. As the song says, "too hot not to cool down." The newness wore off and the euphoric feeling started to becomes painful when the relationship did not fulfill her emotional need for long-term comfort and companionship. In the beginning she didn't feel that was necessary, or maybe she deluded herself into believing he would get a divorce sooner rather than later.

After about a year of enjoying this passionate distraction, she decided that she needed to talk with her therapist, who she had stopped seeing when she met her knight in shining armor. When the relationship came to a screeching halt for various mutual reasons, all the feelings of losing her husband were stirred up once again. But letting go of her lover almost seemed worse, because he was still alive, yet no longer in her life. Even though he offered a port in the storm, it was still her port and the only one on her mind.

Was she ready to let go of this physical, emotional life raft? After running through a gamut of emotions she returned to her therapist. On the day that the relationship blew up she called her therapist for an emergency visit. Although the decision to end it was mutual, it was still very painful and was like another death to her. Even though he was still alive, it almost felt worse than the loss of her husband. She asked herself whether she was just reliving and re-enacting her husband's passing.

She asked her therapist if the she thought that after a year she could still be going through her grieving and healing process. After all she was a fire sign and she usually did things fast. It shouldn't take this long. At least not her mind. Of course the answer was yes, absolutely!

Everyone has their own time frame and ways of dealing with their loss. Sometimes we feel that we are perfectly fine, and we are, but then there is a trigger. For Zoe it was the rollercoaster ride with her lover, but despite all that it was an enjoyable and satisfying distraction. It played a major role in her healing journey until she decided it was no longer serving her, and the pain was outweighing the pleasure.

> Everyone has their own time frame and ways of dealing with their loss.

It just so happened that Venus, the planet that rules love and our relationships, was stationed retrograde during this time. When Venus is retrograde, people tend to reevaluate their relationships and what is really important to them in their relationship. What do they really want? What are they willing to compromise about or not compromise? If they are in a relationship that no longer serves them, they are more open and willing to let it go—which is exactly what Zoe did during this retrograde cycle.

She cut her emotional and physical ties from this man to whom she had bared her soul, her heart and her body. She was no longer willing to live with and accept the idea that he may never change his circumstances and leave his wife, no matter how unhappy he proclaimed himself to be.

Life is too short she said. "I've seen too many of my friends and their husbands leave." She made the decision that she was ready to continue her healing journey but in a different direction.

After all, she reasoned, there is no such thing as a void in life. When one door closes, another one opens. The hard part is being willing to close that first door, and having the faith that another one will indeed open.

Several months after her decision to let go of her illusion she met a wonderful man. Although he was not perfect, he wasn't married. They enjoyed spending time together and they shared many of the same interests. All the stars were aligned and everything at first appeared to be a perfect match.

He was everything she thought she could have hoped for, except for one small detail . . . she wasn't in love with him. The chemistry just wasn't there. She said that she made a conscious decision to once again enjoy peace with herself and enjoy her own space and company.

Zoe later shared with me that she had heard that her friend eventually did get a divorce and relocated to another state.

RETURN TO ROCK 'N' ROLL

Liza had always been a rock 'n' roll junky. She was born and raised in Detroit listening to Motown music. Rock 'n' roll was always her passion. She enjoyed and found refuge in it like it was her garden sanctuary.

After a long debilitating illness with COPD her husband passed away and left her to find herself again. Her life was now to begin as a single woman, living alone for the very first time ever in her life. She had gone from her parents' home to her first marriage that produced two children. That life ended when she divorced after 14 years.

Not too long after her divorce she met Jim, the love of her life. Little did she know that his life was going to be limited due to his heavy smoking habit and poor health choices.

Music and dancing were always important to her because it gave her life energy. After Jim passed away she reconnected with rock 'n' roll, which had been a centering force in her life while growing up in Detroit.

Leon Russell was always her heartthrob and her number one musician to follow. After her husband's passing, she reconnected with her love and passion for rock music and Leon Russell. She began going to his concerts wherever she could see him performing, buying his music, collecting photographs, videos, and artwork. She bought T-shirts with his name and image and decorated them with musical symbols which satisfied her need for creativity and fed her soul.

She had been a graphic artist before marrying Jim and was always a creative person until his illness. Her creativity began to blossom again through her music and her gardening. She found peace and solace in her beautiful garden filled with images of blue birds which she collected in remembrance of him. He had always enjoyed the sight of bluebirds in the garden. She kept her love alive through music and her time in the garden.

She actually keeps a little glass blue bird in every room of her house so she feels his energy when she walks into the room.

I found it interesting when she brought up the need for security in her home and surroundings. I can recall that very same feelings after both of my husbands passed away. The first time, my brother-in-law came in changed all the locks in my house and double bolted the doors. I would lie in bed and think that I heard noises. I preferred not to drive at night. I was very paranoid for a while.

Liza said she notified the local police that she lived alone and asked them to keep an eye on her house when making their patrol in her area. Again, I could recall doing the very same thing.

When Tony passed away I lived in a very secure condominium so I felt safe. But I did look in my rear view mirror before I would put my garage door down to make sure no one was lurking behind me.

But the lost sense of security was balanced by an increase in a sense of freedom. Liza also shared her feeling of growth and independence, in that for the very first time in her adult life she was living alone and didn't have to consider anyone else. She didn't have to cook or clean for anyone but herself, or even get dressed in the morning if she didn't want to. Not that she stopped doing these things, she just did them in her own time and space.

She grew to appreciate and value her independence, which became a valuable commodity to her. Life had taken a new shape and meaning. She had found her "new normal." Although she loved her husband unconditionally and had a good marriage—he treated her like a queen—he was gone now and she had to sprout her own wings and make a new life for herself. She was happy with where and who she was in this new normal she had crafted.

"It's not that I wouldn't welcome another man into my life," she said. "I just don't need a man to make me happy."

It took time but she did reinvent herself. And she is enjoying her new invention.

DRUGS

I guess we could say that drugs come in many forms. This is Hanna's story:

When I spoke with Hanna I was surprised to learn that her husband passed away in September of 2015, which was only three months after my husband passed. Hanna's husband's lung cancer was diagnosed 14 months prior to that, which is when she said she started mourning. He was a musician and a heavy smoker. They were married for 37 years.

When I asked what she did after he died, she said she got trashed with a buddy who was a very good longtime friend of hers and her husband.

She said she felt a surge of energy for about three months after her husband passed away. She felt like she was in high gear and driven to get things done. I could relate to that. I recalled having that same feeling—although I didn't get trashed. It seems that all the people I talked with, especially those who lost a spouse, mentioned that same thing, an adrenalin rush you might say. Perhaps it comes from necessity. There is so much that needs to be done—from the paper work surrounding the spouse's passing, to cleaning out the garage and the closets.

Another thing she noticed was that she stopped watching TV after her husband died. She hated the commercials and was depressed by the news. I can remember feeling that way too, which I thought was very interesting and a little surprising. One of her friends called her to tell her to get ready for the hurricane and she said, "What hurricane?" I could relate to that sense of isolation.

On the plus side, she overcame a lot of her fears and hang ups. She got over her fear of driving over bridges and on interstate highways. Maybe it was because she had no choice if she wanted to go anywhere in the car, but maybe a new kind of courage was being born in her.

Her best and most healing decision was to reconnect with her love for theater.

A friend came over and helped her clean out the garage, which is where she and her husband spent a great deal of their time because it was where her husband smoked. She said she didn't drink while he was sick but she made up for it right after he died. That day cleaning out the garage was a good opportunity to get a little tipsy.

And then something very interesting happened. Michael, a musician and longtime friend of both her and her husband, connected with her about six weeks after her husband passed away. Michael was 17 years younger than her and was separated from his wife. He was exactly what she needed to help her through that very emotional and difficult transition. The sex was exhilarating and a wonderfully welcome distraction from all of the mourning and sadness she had been going through. She felt like a cloud had been lifted from over her head.

Then, something unimaginable happened. About four months after they stared seeing each other, which was very comforting, he went up north to help take care of his ailing father. While he was there, he had a massive heart attack and died at forty-five years old. Needless to say she was devastated.

It wasn't very long after this horrible news that Barney, a high school classmate of her husband who lived across the state, connected with her. She had first met him at her husband's twentieth high school reunion. They started dating, which lasted about a year. She admitted it wasn't a particularly good relationship. They really didn't have much in common, but the sex was a useful salve for her tattered emotions—a temporary band-aide and a great distraction after all that she had been through.

Perhaps her best and most healing decision was to reconnect with her love for theater a few months after her husband passed away. She had always been very active in the music ministry at her church while her husband was alive, and had done a good deal of community theater when she was in her twenties, including having the lead role in several plays.

Getting back into theater was a wonderful outlet for her. It gave her something positive to focus on and gave her structure in her life, which she desperately needed. As was the case with me and many of the caregivers who I spoke with, she felt that she lost her job when her husband died. There was a tremendous void in her life.

And the theater is where she met the love of her life, Matthew. Matt was tall and handsome in her eyes. They had so much in common—theater, religion, music, food. She felt really alive again and it wasn't just about the sex. It was the total package. It was a healthy relationship. It was a relationship where they could both grow and enjoy a full life together.

Although Michael was a musician like her husband, there was the age difference to deal with and he died suddenly. She never really had that much in common with Barney, except for the physical connection, and now she had found someone who was the total package that was right for her.

She shared with me that he got up in front of the entire congregation at their church after she finished singing and proposed to her. And of course she said yes!

Sex and Death ... are they related?

So after doing several interviews, I started asking myself if there is some identifiable connection between sex and death. I know that in astrology there is a connection between the planets in the area of the chart that rules sex and death, but is there a psychological connection?

So I called the therapist who I had gone to see for my bereavement counseling and asked her if there was any research she was aware of to bear this out.

She said that there is a hormonal release when we have sex that makes us feel good. This could also help relieve and speed up the healing process—or at least provide a great distraction. The endorphins that are connected with sex can help elevate our spirits in the short run.

It's very similar to the endorphins that are released when we exercise. People say they get high on exercising. They also get high while having sex.

So I guess the moral to the story is that if you can't have sex, you can at least exercise. I found that it always worked for me, which is why I started doing triathlons after my first husband passed away in 1993 and have continued to maintain a faithful exercise regimen ever since.

*"We are the sum total of our experiences.
Those experiences—be they positive or
negative—make us the person we are, at any
given point in our lives."* — B.J. Neblett

Chapter Fourteen

THOUGHTS MAKE MAGICAL THINGS HAPPEN

I have said several times now that I've always believed there is no such thing as coincidence. The older I get, the more I see and appreciate the magic some people call synchronicity. It's not just that an extremely improbable "coincidence" occurs in a life, it's that the occurrence speaks deeply to the person in some important way—a kind of revelation of who you are. Maybe another way of explaining this is that you attract what you think about, as Ernest Holmes and Willis Kinnear wrote in, *Thoughts Are Things*, which is why it is always important to have productive, healthy thoughts.

Thoughts become manifestations. Everything that happens begins with a thought. I can recall thinking after my husband passed away that I wanted to get involved in some type of volunteer work. My first adventure volunteering was working one afternoon a week as a receptionist in my church office. That was okay for about a month, but then I started to lose enthusiasm. Something always seemed to come up that I needed or preferred to do on my volunteer days.

I finally realized that perhaps this was not the type of volunteer work that I was meant to do. So, I had to come up with something else. I thought about volunteering one morning a week at the hospital gift store. A friend of mine organizes the volunteers at the store and she invited to me to sign up. But once again I had to make a commitment for a specific day and time every week. I felt fairly sure that, as happened with the church office, other things would come and get in the way. I guess that's why I never wanted to go back to a 9-5 job after I was able to get away from it.

That's probably one of the many reasons why my work as an astrological counselor and author has suited me so well all these years.

I couldn't help thinking about my own mother when I walked into the room.

Which brings me to my next "magical thing." While exhibiting at an event one evening, I met a representative from one of the assisted living retirement homes in my area. When she suggested that I might come and do a program for their residents, the idea grabbed me. This could be the volunteer work I was searching for that would feed my soul. I was excited about it in a way I never felt with the other volunteer positions. I could schedule the program at my convenience and I wasn't committed to a weekly schedule and time commitment. And I would be doing something that I love to do. I would be entertaining and sharing my passion. I would be giving these people something else to think about—at least for a while. My plan was to help brighten their day.

So my first program was scheduled and presented to a room full of very senior citizens. I couldn't help but thinking about my own mother when I walked into the room. She always enjoyed social activities and a room full of people. And she always enjoyed my talks when she was able to attend. She was my biggest fan. She came to my first book signing and was so proud of me.

I got so much more of what I wanted as a volunteer from sharing my programs at the nursing homes and retirement centers.

It was such a pleasure to interact with the residents and see their faces light up as I talked about their sun signs and the lunar phases. I shared with them some basics on how the lunar cycle affects our emotions and how people tend to be more emotional when there is a full moon. I loved seeing their faces light up as they realized that they had felt this full moon effect themselves.

Although most of them may not have grasped everything I was saying, I noticed that when I talked about their particular sun sign they would perk up and pay attention. They even began to ask me questions about their children's sun signs.

It seems that everyone enjoys hearing about their sun sign, even if they are in an assisted living facility or a nursing home and have never really thought about astrology before. I certainly enjoyed sharing that information with them.

MORE MAGIC—SPEAKING TO AN ADDICTION GROUP

One evening when I was attending a Chamber of Commerce after hours gathering, I was delighted when a woman pulled me aside and said she wanted to talk with me. I always wear my *Kelly Lowe, Astrological Counselor & Author* name badge when I attend business functions, so she knew who I was and what I did.

I soon learned that she was an addiction counselor who worked for a center in the area. This information brought a smile to my face and if I had been thinking quicker I might have said, "of course you are." Again, I was ready and open to attracting volunteer work but hadn't quite found my niche. But it happened that I had been working with several clients who have struggled with addiction. The thought entered my mind that I would like to be invited to speak to one of the rehab groups. Although I never really pursued the idea, it was very much in the back of mind. Remember, "thoughts are things" that do manifest.

So, back to the woman at the chamber social—the law of attraction, or good fortune worked out once again. She wanted to talk with me about coming to speak to her group. Would I, by any chance, be interested? I told her that not only was I interested, I would be honored to do it.

Opening myself to volunteering was opening me to becoming a new person, changed from the person I was before my husband became ill, and certainly from the person I had to be after he passed.

The universe was giving me new opportunities that were lifting me up and adding on to who I am, like a building rising up story after story.

As B.J. Neblett wrote in his book *Quotable Quotes*,

"We are the sum total of our experiences. Those experiences—be they positive or negative—make us the person we are, at any given point in our lives. And, like a flowing river, those same experiences, and those yet to come, continue to influence and re-shape the person we are, and the person we become. None of us are the same as we were yesterday, nor will be tomorrow."

*"Any motion whatsoever beats inertia,
because inspiration will always be drawn
to motion."* — Elizabeth Gilbert

Chapter Fifteen

VOLUNTEER!

I just gave two examples where I was able to volunteer my skills as an astrological counselor to bring some joy to others along with myself. But the area in which you volunteer need not be anything at which you are skilled—just something you enjoy.

One of the first things I did after Tony passed away was to sign up as a volunteer at golf tournaments. I had often thought during our marriage about doing that, but didn't want to take the time away from "us" to go off and spend several days volunteering.

As Elizabeth Gilbert wrote in her book *Big Magic, Creative Living Beyond Fear*, "Any motion whatsoever beats inertia, because inspiration will always be drawn to motion. Go walk the dog, go pick up every bit of trash on the street outside your home, go walk the dog again, go bake a peach cobbler, go paint some pebbles with brightly colored nail polish and put them in a pile. Make something. Do something. Do anything."

Although she is referring to developing your creativity I also believe and have found that this is a great antidote for grief and coping with a loss. I chose to become more actively involved by volunteering at golf tournaments. Although this may not be everyone's cup of tea, it helped me to fight back the tears.

Tony and I enjoyed attending many professional golf tournaments together over the years. When I first met him, I was a neophyte to golf. I knew nothing. I actually knew less than nothing because what I thought I knew was all wrong! But since he was such an avid golfer it seemed like a fun thing to learn to do. So I decided to learn the game and started taking lessons.

Yes, it is frustrating at first, and can be a frustrating game in general, but it's also wonderful and exhilarating when you get a good shot and see the ball rising and sailing down the fairway. And there's **I was spreading my wings as I was growing and healing.** always that hole in one to look forward to—which I'm still looking forward to but not giving up hope. I was playing with a gal when she did get a hole in one and that was very exciting for everyone in our foursome. Maybe I'm next!

My first golf related volunteer job was at the LPGA course in Daytona Beach, a home course for the Ladies Professional Golf Association. The event was the Symetra Tour Championship. The Symetra tour is a national, professional, women's golf tour that calls itself the "road to the LPGA." Top performers on the Symetra qualify for the "big tour," so this is serious business for the golfers. I drove a golf cart taking the players and their caddies from one hole to the next, which was fun. Some of gals were very chatty and others very serious and quiet. But they were all very pleasant.

The weather was great, and I was out enjoying the fresh air which took my mind off my loss. It was something I had never done before. It was a part of my healing and growth process. I was all about doing new and different things and enjoying new experiences.

I was spreading my wings as I was growing and healing. After working the women's qualifying tournaments a couple of times, I decided to branch out into golf's big league.

My husband and I had visited the Torrey Pines golf course in La Jolla, California, years ago. Although we weren't able to play golf there at the time, we always thought that we would someday. They have two beautiful and challenging courses. We always enjoyed watching the men's Professional Golf Association (PGA) Farmers Open tournament on TV. It is played Torrey Pines every February. TV does not do the courses justice. They are much more beautiful than they appear on TV.

So after putting a few local LPGA tournaments in my resume, I decided to be brave and sign up online to volunteer at this major event. My husband had passed away in June and the tournament was the following February, so it gave me something to look forward to. Having "something to look forward to" is always good. And traveling was at the top of my list of things to do during that first year. That is, as soon as I recovered from my hip replacement. (Yes, I had a hip replacement two months after my husband passed away. But that's another story!)

Since my aunt and uncle lived in San Diego, this trip would be a double pleasure. I planned to go out and have a nice visit with them and enjoy the new experience of volunteering at a major PGA tournament. Life was good.

But wait a minute before you start to envy me. When I arrived for my assigned volunteer job, I discovered that it wasn't exactly what I thought it was going to be.

You see, I signed up online through the volunteer sight to be a "shuttle driver," which is what the job was called that I did at the LPGA tournament in Florida. As it turned out the "shuttle" I had signed up for at the PGA tournament meant I was to drive players to and from the San Diego Airport.

I said "are you kidding me?" I don't drive on the California Freeways. Everyone knows they are notorious and only the locals dare risk it. It seems that I totally misunderstood the description of the job on the website. I thought shuttle meant driving the players around the golf course like I did for the LPGA tournament in Florida—a great way to spend the day—not battling the tense jam-ups of California freeway traffic.

As it turned out the only player shuttles that are used at Torrey Pines are to take the golfers from the practice putting green area to the practice driving range at the top of a big long hill. This is the job that I wanted, that I thought I was signing up for in the first place.

I guess if I had been a local resident that would have been the end of it. They'd have said "tough luck Kelly, maybe next year." But when they learned I had flown all the way from Florida to volunteer at this event, they said they'd see what they could do about getting me into the inner, closed circle that drove the players from the putting green to the practice range. It seems that committee is pretty tight and made up of people who've worked together for years. I was told it is very tough to get a spot as a "golf cart shuttle" driver.

But as luck, or God would have it, I was able to meet with the chairman who was in charge of that team of volunteers and he managed to fit me into their schedule. So I got to meet and drive the big name golfers around, and watch them practice up close. Unfortunately Phil Mickelson didn't ride the shuttle. He used his personal cart and driver. It was a memorable experience but would have been more memorable if I had gotten to drive Phil. I did get to watch him finish his round on Friday, but he didn't score well enough in the first two rounds to make the cut and go on to play the weekend that year.

The weather was perfect the days that I worked, but it turned very nasty the last day of the tournament—which I was not scheduled to work, thankfully. They had to suspend play and finish on Monday. That was the year that a horrific storm came through and uprooted many of the beautiful trees, totally changing the terrain and appearance of the course.

The weather in La Jolla that time of winter, which is always when the "Farmer's Open" is played, can be beautiful or terrible. And sometimes it's both on any given day. That's California in February.

When my aunt asked me if I was coming back the following year to volunteer for the event, I told her that once was enough. It was a wonderful and memorable experience. I got a very nice hat, golf shirt and windbreaker as a part of my registration fee, which I am continuing to enjoy. I totally appreciated and enjoyed the experience, but I wouldn't ask my aunt and uncle to make the morning commute to La Jolla again. The traffic was ... well, I'll just say you have to experience it to know what I mean.

And while I'm at it, I'll just say thank you Aunt Jeannie and Uncle Frank for all that you have done and do for me. I couldn't have made it thought that first year without you. I would add that when any of us are recovering from loss it isn't easy to let people get near enough to see our pain—even when they are close family. I was glad I resisted that impulse. Seeing other hearts filled with compassion can be our invitation back into the world.

Although this was a trip of a lifetime for me— to be a volunteer at this major PGA Tournament— It was bittersweet. I always thought that I would be watching this tournament with Tony. But I felt that working at that tournament was one of the turning points in my healing journey. At some moment you just have to step off the curb and cross the street alone, without the beloved partner who had helped give life purpose. I felt a full gamut of emotions, as I reflected on our trip to California the first year after we met. We had a wonderful time visiting my aunt and uncle in San Diego and drove up to Torrey Pines to see the golf courses.

Life tends to be a roller coaster during the times of loss and adjustment. There was the anticipation during the flight out there, the disappointment of not having the job that I thought I had signed up for, and sadness of not having Tony there to enjoy watching the tournament with me. Not that he would have been a volunteer—that was not his thing. But he would have enjoyed being a spectator. He so loved golf! That's the thought I held on to as I returned home to Florida.

It takes as long as it needs to take before moving forward after a divorce, the death of a spouse, or any loss. There is no magic formula.

Chapter Sixteen

DIVORCE AND THE TOLL OF NEW BEGINNINGS

Opportunities for change and growth come in many forms. Of course the most final is when a spouse or loved one passes on, but a divorce is also a loss—especially if it was not your idea. Oftentimes, there is a victim and a villain when there is a divorce (and there might be disagreement over which is which).

The divorcee or divorcer is still around. The feelings may linger for an extended period of time. There may always be the thought that you could get back together, or guilt about what you could have done to save the marriage Death, on the other hand, is very final.

In the 2005 academy award winning movie *Sideways*, which I saw during a girls night out at our local Cinematique, we enjoyed the adventurous trip through the Santa Barbara wine region by two buddies—a handsome soon-to-be-married actor Jack Cole, played by Thomas Haden Church, and a down-on-his-luck divorcee Miles Raymond, performed by Paul Giamatti.

Although Miles has been divorced for five years, he can't get over his ex-wife. He keeps thinking they are going to get back together again until he runs into her at his friend's wedding—along with her new husband—and finds out that she is pregnant. He finally gets the message and decides it's time to move on. He goes back to the wine country and hooks up with a woman he met there who was very interested in him. It took being slapped in the face by the facts, but he was finally able to move forward with his life.

I think what resonated with me was that it takes as long as it needs to take before moving forward following a divorce, the death of a spouse, or any other loss. There is no magic formula.

Having gone through both a divorce and the loss of two husbands, I could certainly identify with this movie.

* * *

If there is a formula, although probably not a *magic* formula, the closest I have seen is the blog by Family and Marriage Counselor Wendy Crane. With her permission I am sharing her article on transforming one's self after going through divorce. I've summarized the major points here.

In the article she details four steps to a happier you. The first step, Wendy writes, is acknowledging that loneliness is not solved through a relationship with someone else, because, as many of you know, sometimes the deepest loneliness actually occurs within relationship. It is resolved through remembering that your foremost relationship is with Y-O-U! This is the second step. If you are in a partnered relationship, the relationship you develop with yourself will serve to enhance and deepen how you share yourself with your partner.

For the third step, she says to remember we are derived from a much greater source of energy than we could ever imagine, and staying connected with that *source*—which is comprised of *love*—fills the hole within you that we often call "loneliness."

No human person can do that for you. As a great and wise teacher once reminded me: "When you are alone, you are *with yourself*." So, as the fourth step, Wendy says if you want to overcome loneliness, it's time to cozy up with you and only you.

How can I develop a deeper relationship with myself, you ask? Here are 10 ways Wendy Crane says you make it happen:

1. **Listen:** Do you ever notice or hear a little nagging sensation or voice within you that seems to guide you toward the next step in your life? It may nudge you to make a change, try something new, or bring something to a close. It always starts low and subtle and if unacknowledged, can develop into a loud, screaming obstacle that will not move until you choose to pay attention. This is your inner knowing, often called intuition, your soul, or your Truth. Part of strengthening your relationship with yourself is about trusting this inner voice and heeding its call. Become an active and attentive listener to the part of you who seeks your highest good. The more you trust it, the more clear your life path becomes, and the

less opportunity you have to abandon yourself. If you choose to stop abandoning yourself, loneliness dissipates.

2. **Honor and respect your Truth:** These are the actions that follow once you have chosen to listen to and trust your *Self*. If you want others to honor and respect you, you must begin with honoring and respecting *you*. If you consistently throw yourself under the bus, apologize for your existence, or minimize your experience, you deny the truth of who you really are. If you honor and respect what feels true for you, you will set better boundaries, receive more love and feel supported. It is difficult to feel empty when you are taking good care of yourself.

3. **Be patient:** Take it easy on yourself. Rome was not built in a day. Oftentimes, you may have internalized messages or experiences from childhood that cause you to set up walls of protection and patterns of disconnecting from yourself in order to survive. Deconstructing your walls and developing patterns of connection and trust within yourself through the first two steps, can take time and practice. This becomes your "work." This process is often part of the life lessons you are here to learn. Your challenges become your teachers. Take your time to allow the learning to heal you.

4. **Speak up:** Use your words. Tell the truth. Say only what you mean and mean what you say. Do not agree to something that causes your stomach to churn or feel uneasy (that is a clear sign you are surrendering your power and abandoning your-

Kelly Lowe

self). In the speaking of your Truth, you honor yourself and those around you; you develop trust that you can count on yourself to advocate for what you need and ask for what you want. Release fear about expressing yourself—you are worth speaking up for. The more you love and value yourself, the easier it will be for the words to come out.

5. **Develop a spiritual practice:** You come from a great *Source*. What name you call that *Source* is not as important as your relationship with *It*. The relationship between you and your *Source* is what a spiritual practice nurtures. This is where prayer, meditation, yoga, service, time in nature, mindfulness, music, art, and creativity come in. Engage in activities that help you feel connected to something much bigger than you. Practice humility, surrender, and experience grace. When connected to this energy of love, allow it to permeate all of your cells and fill you up. When your whole being is filled with love, it is very difficult to also feel lonely at the same time.

6. **Do something nice:** Just as you would in a traditional relationship, be thoughtful. When there is something that comes up that you know you would like to do, take yourself. Watch the movie that you've been wanting to see, cook foods that nurture you, update your home or wardrobe to match your new outlook, take yourself for a walk or get some extra sleep. This is all about taking care of *yourself*. Identify and give yourself what you need in this moment. Believe that you deserve it and allow yourself to receive.

7. **Hug yourself:** This is another gift to give yourself. It might feel funny at first, but it feels good! Be mindful of what you feel when you give yourself this type of positive attention. Notice how different it might feel from other types of attention—such as judgments, pressure, and self-rejection.

8. **Say "I love you" (A LOT!):** When you are getting ready each morning, take a moment to look into the mirror, look right into your own eyes and say, "I love you, I love you, I love you." Really see yourself, see beyond the surface and all the imperfections, right into your inner-being—the one who tries and who makes mistakes, and who works so hard. And before you go to sleep each night, take one more moment to really see yourself and say, "I love you. Thank you. Tomorrow is a new day." Feel free to add in other times as well. Do this every day for thirty days and notice what happens.

9. **Ask for support:** When you need help, ask. You don't need to create a crisis, drama, get sick or throw a temper tantrum in order to get others to notice that you need help. In listening, speaking up, and honoring your truth, you will know when you need help and will find the words that you need to ask in a clear, concise way.

10. **Play:** When you allow yourself to shed the armor of adulthood for periods of time, you allow that inner-you to come out and play. Get down on the floor and play with a child, run and jump in a park, play with your pet, be silly, laugh, or choose a workout style that is more playground

than machines. Giving yourself permission to play allows you to get in touch with your creativity, vulnerability, and passion. Get to know this part of yourself—it has much to teach you.

It is my personal sincere feeling and believe that this advice is applicable for moving forward after the loss of a spouse through death as well as divorce, as both losses can create a sense of loneliness. Thank you Wendy for allowing me to share . . .

For more helpful information about Divorce Recovery visit Wendy Crane's website. You can download the full article free and find other helpful information. https://www.solflowerwellness.com/divorce-recovery/

> *"Sex and golf are the two things you can enjoy even if you're not good at them."*
> *— Kevin Costner*

CHAPTER SEVENTEEN

SEX OVER 50 IS NOT FOR SISSIES

She was married to her best friend and drinking buddy—someone she could laugh and have a good time with. Then the unexpected hit him. He contracted hepatitis C. He stopped drinking. He stopped smoking. He stopped laughing and they stopped having sex. He became a completely different person. Their life totally changed.

In her mind, he was still her best friend and she was more than willing and happy to take care of him. And after all, she was a Pisces. Of all the zodiac signs, Pisces are perhaps the most inclined to be caregivers, and Virgos are right there with them. That's probably why we find so many of them in the healthcare profession.

Although she had a full time job that was really more than full time, she devoted herself to taking care of this man who had been her husband and best friend for over twenty-one years. She saw him through his darkest days and into his recovery. He beat the hepatitis C with her by his side. She was, by all measures, a compassionate caregiver.

Just about the time she thought the worst was behind her, the unthinkable happened. She was diagnosed with small bowel cancer, which is very rare and very aggressive. The survival rate is less than five percent. I first met Mary when she attended one of my astrology workshops. I had just learned that my husband had been diagnosed with the very same cancer. I couldn't believe it when she approached me after class and told me. What are the chances of that happening?

She shared with me that she had already been through the surgery and treatment and was in remission and doing great. This was very encouraging and gave us a ray of hope. She was one of the very fortunate five percent who had survived. She was very supportive and a good friend through my husband's five-year battle, even though, as it turned out, he was not one of lucky ones—the one in twenty who would survive the cancer.

Unfortunately, when Mary was diagnosed, her husband said he couldn't "do sick." He was not a caregiver and didn't want to be married to her any more. He had met someone else and wanted a divorce.

So her life became an out-of-control roller coaster ride. She felt like she was flailing. She didn't know where to turn, so she threw herself into her work, trying to masque her hurt and disappointment in this man whom she had taken care of during his time of need. Sometimes life just isn't fair and this was certainly one of those times. She was devastated. She was beginning to wonder if the sun was ever going rise again.

Just about the time she had reached the end of her rope, dangling over the pit of despair, a friend told her that she needed to pray about it. She had proven she couldn't handle it on her own so it was time to seek help from a higher source. It made perfect sense to me. Yes, we need to do our own part of the work, but we don't have to do it all. The simple words we so often hear are more than a cliché: "Let go and let God."

So as she was driving home from work one day, her phone rang. It was the higher source calling her. Actually it was her mother who lived in another state telling her that the house next door to hers had become available and suggested she consider moving back to her hometown. She literally picked herself up, dusted herself off and moved back to live next door to her mother.

She was very employable and it didn't take her long to land a nice position in her new location. A new life was being born. As Jimmy Buffett sings, "Changes in Latitude, Changes in Attitude."

Now she is back in her hometown, divorced and on the dating scene at age fifty-three. Dating wasn't new to her, but it certainly was different than when she was thirty-two. She met what she thought was a really nice guy in a neighborhood bar. He was cute and there was definitely a spark between them. They talked for hours the first night they met.

Mary had been given advice from a friend about the things you shouldn't talk about when you meet someone for the first time: Don't talk about your divorce. Don't talk about politics. Don't talk about sex. And don't talk about religion. Of course within twenty minutes they had covered all those subjects.

After four hours of getting to know each other, he walked her to her car, kissed her goodnight and said he was going to call her. He never did. She learned later from someone who had seen them in the bar that he was not the most stable guy in town. So she had dodged the proverbial bullet, avoiding a first post-divorce relationship that was doomed from the start. She never heard from him again.

Maybe there was a better way to meet someone, she thought, and decided to go on *Match.com*. She was motivated. After all, she was only fifty-three and really wanted to meet a nice guy. She actively worked at it, which I've heard is what you really need to do if you're going to date online. You have to check your hits every day and reach out to anyone you think is interesting. It's a numbers game. I actually know a lot of people who have met Mr. or Ms. Right on those sites and ended up happily married to them.

Mary did date one of her "matches" for eighteen months, even though he never told her he loved her—which bothered her. She wanted more, so she finally asked him how he felt about her after all their time together. He said he just wanted to be "friends with benefits." Well, that didn't work for her at this stage in her life.

So, on the heels of their breakup she was working a trade show out of town when she ran into an old friend whom she had known years earlier while she was married to her "best friend." As it turned out, while she was single he was now married—of course unhappily—but married nonetheless. And, of course, there were too many complications, mostly financial, for him to get a divorce.

He was, however, able to help her professionally through his business connections, so they managed to take quite a few trips together. And of course, she fell in love with him to no avail. This lasted about a year before she just couldn't take it anymore. Again, life was too short to be so miserable.

This is when she decided to "order a new one" on the internet. She had a little more experience now and knew what she wanted—and especially what she didn't want. She had kissed a lot of frogs up to this point. She had taken care of her husband through hepatitis C and survived small bowel cancer. She made a major change in her life by moving back to her home town and landing a dynamite job. Now, at age fifty-seven, it was her turn to find happiness with the right man, which is exactly what she did— or thought she had.

Mr. Right had a few flaws in his armor and skeletons in his closet.

She moved back to Florida where she really enjoyed living and went on line with a whole new profile and outlook. She was being very cautious as to what she wanted to attract. She had her priorities in order and after a short search she thought that she had found Mr. Right.

Of course, there's always a few things you'd like to change, but for the most part he was perfect for her. He played the guitar, he was nice looking and funny, and most of all, he adored her. Now she is really enjoying the sunrises.

Unfortunately, Mr. Right had a few flaws in

his armor and skeletons in his closet that took her by surprise. The flaws and incompatibilities started surfacing right around the 90 day mark. In astrology, 90 days is when a new relationship can be expected to move to a different level and take on a different tone or complexion. It either advances into something better where the couple will feel even closer, or they start to drift apart or end it right then.

In this case major health issues were one of the skeletons in his closet. He was not a healthy person, which she learned through several trips to the emergency room. It was not long after their 90-day mark that he made his final trip to the ER. It wasn't until after he passed away that she discovered he was married—separated, but still married. Regardless, Mary grieved his passing and needed time to sort it all out. Fortunately, she was able to benefit from bereavement counseling .

Following her divorce years earlier, Mary never doubted that she would date again. But now, having followed that path through several twists and turns, she could testify that dating after fifty is definitely not for sissies.

So once again she picked herself up, dusted off, and jumped back into her very demanding, high profile job. After all, she told herself, life had been very fulfilling and busy before she met her now departed love. Mary hadn't changed her mind about love, nor did she harbor regrets. She still believed it is more fun to have someone to share sunrises and sunsets with. She hadn't given up on meeting Mr. Right on a dating sight, but decided to take a break, knowing that the sun always rises. Who knows, Mr. Right could show up on one of her sunrise beach walks.

*In my practice and in my personal life,
I've seen the path many friends and clients
have traveled as they dealt with loss.*

Chapter Eighteen

OTHER VOICES, OTHER STORIES

CONVERSATIONS WITH WOMEN WHO HAVE FOUND THEIR "NEW NORMAL"

I learned a long time ago during an astrology reading I had with by Noel Tyl, a prominent astrologer and author, that I needed structure in my life. He told me many things during that reading, but the real jewel and most memorable was that I needed structure in my life. For those of you who speak the language, I was born with Saturn on my ascendant, which I have found to be a blessing in times of stress or distress throughout my life's journey.

So when *push comes to shove* and the *(you-know-what) hits the fan,* as my daddy—a retired Navy man—used to say, I find solace, security, and comfort in planning and organizing a structured life. The first time I was widowed, I started training for triathlons. That would be mini-triathlons of course, half-mile swim, twelve-mile bike ride, and three-mile run. But still, at fifty years old that wasn't too shabby. It made me feel good about myself and helped me grow physically and emotionally stronger to deal with my loss.

I also immersed myself in my work. I began seeing clients again, teaching and doing workshops again. And I taught an astrology course at the local college. I enjoyed living a very structured and fulfilling life. But then, I remembered and knew that was true from my reading with Noel Tyl. That was exactly what feeds my soul and could be counted on to help me grow strong again.

So when I was once again widowed, after the initial shock I dug down deep to reconnect with what I needed to do to find my "new normal." Yes, even if you know the person is not going to survive their illness, there is still a period of shock when they make their transition. So once I had regained some sense of balance, I became very structured in my workout routine. I did not see any more triathlon training in my future, but I did join a new gym which offered more classes and equipment in addition to the Olympic size pool I had been enjoying at the YMCA.

Once again, I immersed myself in my work and increased my schedule of doing workshops and seeing clients. Since I had written my first book during my husband's chemo treatment and recovery, I decided this was the time for me to allow the new book growing inside me to come out into the light of day. Everything I had experienced since writing *An Astrologer's Journey* was making me stronger, feeding my soul, and giving me a level of wisdom I hadn't known before.

As I began imagining the new book in conferences with my editor, I also branched out in my local community. I joined and became active in my local Chamber of Commerce. I joined the Yacht Club, where I grew excited about resuming my astrological talks there which I called "Dinner with the Stars." I joined the local Travel and Ski Club. Although I am no longer able to ski, it was a great social outlet and helped to reconnect with that community.

Loss in Our Time or Our Time of Life

In my practice and in my personal life, I've seen the path many friends and clients have traveled as they dealt with loss. Sometimes I am able to help them, and on many occasions I have learned from their experiences. It seemed like there was a lot of that—meaning recovery from loss— going around at about the same time my husband passed. And of course I started to energetically attract clients who were going through the same thing.

I learned through our conversations what it was that they did to feed their souls in those challenging times in order to move toward with their new normal. What helped them to grow and find themselves again after their loss? I've added their revelations to those I experienced myself.

Reinvention Goes More than Skin Deep

Joann was always very active in her church, so when her husband, Jim, developed Parkinson's and passed away after seven years of her lovingly caring for him, it was only natural for her to become even more involved in her church. She said she found comfort and strength in her connection with God. Without her faith she could not have made it

---

through. She knew in her heart that he was home again with Jesus and he would no longer be suffering. This was a certainty in her heart and mind, and it gave her solace.

Although she was free of the considerable care Jim required every day, like many caregivers before her, she had a hard time embracing this as freedom. Instead, she felt that she had lost her job and purpose after Jim's passing. She set about finding a "new normal" that didn't include caring for Jim. She first joined a bereavement group at her church to help her through the initial shock—and she stopped doing things that no longer suited or served her.

She was involved in a direct marketing company that was very time consuming and unrewarding, but she had been inspired to work at it while Jim was battling his disease. She let go of that and soon found a niche, a purpose that fed her soul and was more rewarding. She and Jim had been greyhound rescue parents for years, but when they lost their dog Bo during Jim's illness, they decided not to adopt another greyhound. It was just too much in addition to taking care of her husband.

Then, about a year after Jim's passing, she became a foster parent to Lizzie, a three-legged greyhound who she ended up adopting. In addition to making Lizzie her own, she accidently fell into becoming a pet sitter, which has truly been her niche and calling. It started with friends and neighbors and grew into a full scale business which she loves and is very good at.

Oh yes, not very long after her loss she decided to have some cosmetic surgery which took twenty years off of her appearance. Now that's what I call reinventing yourself and finding the "new normal."

Finally, she has become a facilitator for the bereavement group at her church. She said she gets so much more than she gives and this truly feeds her soul and spirit.

SYLVIA'S STORY: BELIEVE THAT ANYTHING IS POSSIBLE

Sylvia and her husband Gene owned and operated a health and fresh produce store in my neighborhood. The store is on my way home from my morning rituals at the gym. I enjoyed stopping a couple days a week and visiting with them while picking up my vitamin supplements or anything else I needed to help address any issues that that might be affecting my body at the time. And their fresh produce are the best—much better than my local chain supermarket.

Not only were they warm and friendly, hardworking and caring people, they were very knowledgeable in homeopathic and natural remedies. They were always willing to take time to listen and assist customers with whatever remedies they could offer. I can remember one morning talking to Gene about being awake all night with leg cramps. He immediately directed me to the some magical potion of apple cider vinegar, natural ginger, and garlic juice. It tasted horrific, but oh my God, did it ever work!

That's just one of the many times Gene came to my rescue. He was a natural at helping people and anyone who knew him couldn't help but love him.

TRANSITION

Right around the time that my husband was going through his cancer treatment, I walked into their store one day and learned that Gene had also been diagnosed with cancer and was going through treatment. I had thought he looked to be losing weight and was a little fragile, but you would never have known it by his attitude. He was still as warm, friendly, and caring as he had always been.

Even after his treatments began, whenever I asked how he was doing he would always say "great." He was optimistic, positive and always showed the appearance of beating it. But he was looking more and more frail as time progressed, until finally one day he was no longer able to come into the store.

Family members started pitching in to help keep the doors open while Sylvia, Gene's wife, was spending more and more time with him at home. And then hospice was called in. I kept asking about him, knowing that one day I was going to get the bad news. It finally came about nine months after my husband had passed away.

I felt awful for Sylvia and the family. Not only did she lose her husband, but she had a business to try to save. She had to make a living. As anyone knows who has lost someone, especially a spouse, things begin to change as soon as the diagnosis is delivered. And when you're trying to make a living and run a business along with dealing with the illness, it can be overwhelming. But somehow they managed to keep the doors open.

When I spoke with Sylvia I could see and feel that she had a strong spirit and faith. She was determined. She told me her faith in God—and a life beyond this one—is what saved her. She said she felt close to Gene when she was at the store.

The "vultures" starting circling immediately after the news got around that she was now a widow struggling with a business. Although she didn't want to sell the store, she was being encouraged to let it go. The struggle with Gene's illness and passing had no doubt set the business back. But the store was still a part of Gene, and she did not want to let go of it.

She and Gene had been married for 33 years. They met while working at an A&P grocery store. Over the years they had owned and operated several different businesses together, so she was not a foreigner to the hard work that it takes to run a small business. And she was a person with a good head for business. Although she had all these things going for her and did not want to let the store go, she was talked into listing it with a realtor. Almost immediately after Gene passed a lowball offer came in. She was sick about it, but encouraged to accept, which she reluctantly did. She wasn't thinking clearly, but down deep in her heart of hearts, she knew she wanted to keep the store. She prayed about whether she should follow through with the sale.

Once again Sylvia's faith came through for her.

Sylvia has a very strong faith. She said that in her life, "God has first place." She has read the bible all the way through twice, but is not a bible thumping kind of a person who demands that you see things her way. When I asked her about her religious beliefs, she said, "Religion is man's idea of God's expectations of us." She believes that the most important thing is to, "Love God, love yourself and love your fellow man—and with this all things are possible."

She shared this passage from the bible with me. She has memorized the words and repeats them every day. She said this has gotten her through losing Gene.

Proverbs 3:5,6
5. Trust in the Lord with all your heart and
lean not on your own understanding:
6. In all your ways acknowledge Him,
and He shall direct your paths.

Her prayers and faith were answered. As it turned out the offer to buy the business did not go through for various reason which I will not go into. But in her heart of hearts Sylvia knew that her prayers had been answered. She told the realtor to take the store off the market. She knew she had a lot of work and praying to do to get the store back on its feet and to catch up on the bills. It was a struggle, and without family, friends and the community pulling together to help her, she could not have made it.

Then just about the time she was beginning to see the light of day, seven months after Gene passed away, Hurricane Matthew hit us. It flooded the store. The entire community was pretty devastated by the storm. It was sad for me to drive down the street and see all the store fronts boarded up.

But once again Sylvia's faith came through for her. She knew that God was going to take care of her, and he did.

Someone told her about FEMA, the Federal Emergency Management Agency, the government organization that helps small businesses after a natural disaster, as well as homeowners. She had to apply by filling out tons of paperwork and jumping through a series of hoops, which she was willing to do. The love that she and Gene shared, and the passion they both felt for the health food business, kept her going. The business was a part of Gene and she did not want to let it go. And she believed that God was with her every step of the way. And so, it turned out, he was.

With the help of her FEMA loan and the support of her family, friends and community, she was able to get the store up and running once again. She and her "team" personally repainted, redecorated, redid the floors, and generally revitalized the store. As a regular customer I can attest that the store and Sylvia are going stronger than ever. Once again, her faith had seen her through.

A CONSCIOUS DECISION TO MOVE FORWARD—
NO ONE CAN DO IT FOR YOU.

Lisa had always been a very self-sufficient, independent lady. She enjoyed cooking, sewing, gardening, reading, and always allowed time to keep up with her tan by the pool. She especially enjoyed her pets. She always had a dog and a cat to care for, and when she met Bill after being divorced for nine years, he fit into her life perfectly. He was a gem. She enjoyed and appreciated the wonderful relationship that they had together. They enjoyed traveling together, going out on Friday nights and knowing they could talk together about anything. For Lisa, having Bill to bounce her ideas off was wonderful.

When he passed away after a long battle with prostate cancer, she was devastated. Due to family circumstance and complications, she was forced to sell their home. Her life was going to change drastically.

After selling her house in the city, she started a new life in the "country," near where her very good friends lived. She told me she had made a conscious decision to move forward. "No one else can do it for you," she said.

At 72 years old she chose to start a new life in a new place and moved to a small retirement community And who would have thought that she would meet a very special, wonderful man there. It had been two and a half years since her significant other had passed away, when one evening she was at a dance with a girlfriend whose husband was out of town. It was a perchance fluke that Lisa was even there that night. She had never before been to the dances that happened on a regular basis at the new community, but thought "why not" when her girlfriend invited her.

It just so happened that sitting across from her that evening was a very nice looking, interesting gentlemen who asked her to dance. She quickly found out that it was also his first time at one of the dances. His wife had passed away two months prior and it was the first time he had been out to a social event. They enjoyed a delightful evening, and he invited her to dinner the next evening—which led to them spending a lot more time together.

She soon learned that he was a devout, traditional Catholic who believed that having sex out of wedlock was a sin. She, on the other hand, was not really into traditional religion. Was this to be the deal breaker? No, not really . . .

Who would have thought that she, now 74 years old, and he, at 81, would once again find love. After almost a year of dating and spending a lot of time together they decided they wanted to spend the rest of whatever time they had left on this earth together. I guess the moral to this story—and reason they wanted to share it—is that we're never too old to find love and have a relationship, if that is what we want. She shared with me that she now goes to church with him—which was something that really surprised me!

"Where attention goes energy flows. What you place your attention on blossoms and blooms, and what you drift your attention away from withers, diminishes and dies"
— Davidji

CHAPTER NINETEEN

THE 2ND YEAR ANNIVERSARY, LIFE CONTINUES

The first anniversary of Tony's passing was spent visiting family in California and then on to the spiritual Qigong retreat in Hawaii I have shared with you. I wanted to just escape and run away for the first anniversary and in many ways that was exactly what I needed to do. And as fate would have it, the retreat became a springboard into the rest of my life.

But the second anniversary was different. I chose to stay home in the home that Tony and I had shared. I wanted to embrace and acknowledge his impact and blessings in my life and the lives of his family.

So when I extended the invitation to our family to gather for a cookout at our home, it was unanimously accepted. They too wanted to celebrate and acknowledge the major role that he had played in our lives.

We laughed, we told stories, we looked at pictures, we remembered the good times we shared with him. His sister Linda, who had known him the longest, of course had the best stories. But her most cherished memories were about our trips to Las Vegas together. She explained that she never sits down at a blackjack table without hearing her brother say, "Linky, (his nickname for her) you gotta take a hit on 16 . . ." She loved her big brother, as we all did.

My life is certainly different after moving forward through the first two years following Tony's passing. It was a journey that only I could travel with myself and for myself. I carried with me all the wonderful memories which I cherished, along with the company of my family and friends who are very near and dear to me.

As I spoke with other widows, I discovered that many of them felt the same way that I did. They did not feel that they needed another man in their life to make them happy. They were happy and content in their own space. If someone absolutely wonderful came along they might reconsider, but they were not hitting the bars or doing *Match.com*—not that there is anything wrong with that. It just didn't suit the needs for the woman I spoke with. Most of them were enjoying doing their own thing in their own way, just as I had learned to do.

> My list was specific about what and who I wanted to attract.

After my husband Larry passed away in 1992, I made myself a list of what I wanted in a relationship. Some of the things remained the same when Tony passed away in 2015, and some were very different. The list was definitely longer. I called it my "intention list." I set my intentions with the energy of a "new moon," exactly as I have taught and described in my chapter about using the lunar cycles. My list was specific about what and who I wanted to attract.

I kept the list next to my bed so I could re-read it on every new moon and reevaluate to make changes or updates. I have always found this to be a positive way to manifest my desires. I tried to be as specific and detailed as possible. In addition to my list, I prayed that when the time was right and my heart was ready, the right man would come into my life again and I would be ready to appreciate him.

Although that is certainly not a priority for me at this time in my life—and my intentions list keeps evolving—I always keep an open mind and continue to enjoy every sunrise.

One never knows where you might meet someone. It's usually when you least expect it, but I believe it is important to set your intentions, as with everything in life.

I can recall many years ago, when I was a young woman, reading *The Power of Positive Thinking* by Norman Vincent Peale. Unfortunately the copy with all my handwritten notes did not make it through my many moves over the years, but the message I took from the book has remained. As I worked my way deeper into an understanding of astrological influences, I became even more convinced of the power of intention and attraction.

As I mentioned earlier, I was also influenced by Ernest Holmes and Willis Kinnear's *Thoughts are Things*, which was published in 1967. As its title suggests, thoughts are things, and we attract what we think about. Our minds are gardens of thoughts and I believe we manifest and grow the seeds that we plant in our minds. So it was no surprise that I was attracted to Davidji's meditations, which take this one step further.

ATTENTION—INTENTION WITH *DAVIDJI*

Within about the first year of Tony's passing, I found a wonderful meditation group close to home. It was through this lovely group of ladies that I was introduced to a smart phone "app" called "Insight Timer."

This is a free app you can get on your phone through which you can select from 7,500 free meditations. Fortunately the ladies in the group had narrowed the field down for me, and I zeroed in on a meditation leader called *Davidji*. So now I make a concerted effort to keep a date with him in my living room every afternoon.

One of my favorite meditations is called "Attention—Intention." *Davidji* leads in by saying . . .

"Where attention goes, energy flows. What you place your attention on blossoms and blooms, and what you drift your attention away from withers, diminishes and dies.

"If we can truly learn that what we place our attention on elevates, and what we drift it from diminishes, then we would never grieve, we would never waste energy. We would never knowingly prolong pain.

"It all comes down to attention. Wherever it is, you are giving, consciously or unconsciously, power to that thing. Intention is a transformational property. Attention activates, intention transforms. When you are able to merge attention with intention, you can create the next unfolding."

So what is it that you would like to manifest into your life? Perhaps you're happy with your life just the way it is, or perhaps you are one of those ready for the next unfolding.

MANIFESTING MY "BUCKET LIST"

A little more than two years after Tony passed, I was attending a local chamber of commerce social event when a friend of mine who is a travel agent was talking about a cruise—a trip to Barcelona that she was organizing. My ears immediately perked up. Barcelona was on my "bucket list."

My friend Ellen and I had been talking about doing this for some time. We were just waiting for a good deal and the right opportunity. And this was it. I immediately called Ellen when I heard about it, and she said yes. We put down our deposit eight months in advance, and the rest became part of my personal history.

My intention was to have a wonderful and memorable trip. Ellen and I had traveled together before, so I knew we were compatible. I must say it was everything I could have possibly imagined it to be.

The cruise would actually depart from Barcelona and we arrived there two days prior to our planned departure. It so happened we arrived during Catalonia's demonstrations for independence, but fortunately they were all peaceful.

After touring Barcelona and enjoying its wonderful food and wine, we boarded our cruise ship. Our first port of call was Naples, Italy. We met our first tour guide and enjoyed a luxurious, comfortable bus ride to Pompeii, where we walked the streets with our guide.

Each day was a new port with a new tour guide as we enjoyed the breathtaking views of the mountainous Amalfi coast in the Salerno province in Southern Italy. To say that driving the Amalfi coast was breathtaking is putting it mildly.

We toured Positano, Sorrento, Vatican City and the ancient Coliseum. We shopped at the leather market in Florence, took pictures of Michelangelo's David and then went on to the Leaning Tower of Pisa, which was not at all what I expected. I was disappointed to find it very commercialized with a lot of vendors as you came through the entrance gates.

No matter where you go, there you are.

Then we went on to Cannes. Fortunately it was not during the big film festival. Monaco was one of my favorite places. We got to see the changing of the guards and the church where Princess Grace and Prince Rainier were married. And of course I was one of those who choose to hike up the mountain to see the famous Monte Carlo Casino. Our tour bus was not permitted in that area so we had to make the trek on foot. I was a little disappointed that I didn't get to gamble in the casino. There just wasn't enough time.

Our last port of call was Palma de Majorca, Spain, a place that I would love to return to and spend more time. This whole experience was a trip of a lifetime for me. The weather was perfect. The food and wine were magnificent and the friends and people that I was able to connect with during the trip were wonderful. The whole experience was everything and more than I could have intended it to be.

The trip of my second anniversary was much different than the meditative retreat that marked the first anniversary after Tony's passing. Had I spent the first anniversary on the cruise it would have left me empty. My needs were different then, as were my intentions and the energy that drew me to Hawaii for the Qigong introduction.

WHAT HAVE THESE TWO YEARS TAUGHT ME?

No matter where you go, there you are. You can run, you can travel the world, but you can't hide from yourself. You can stay busy working, volunteering, taking care of family, cooking and cleaning, watching TV or reading.

These are all among the things that make up a life, but they can be a way to hide from a life. It all depends on whether you are present in each moment. Wherever you go and whatever you are doing, there you are. Be there fully.

So I've come to the conclusion that the first and most important thing in life is to find peace and happiness within—essentially to be happy with yourself and allow yourself to believe it. Enjoy every sunrise. Let each day be a fresh mental start. Remember, no matter how dark any time might feel, *the Sun Always Rises*. Will you believe that it's true, and that you can rise with it?

Yes, some days the sun seems to bring more light than others, but whether it will rise every morning is as certain as my faith that we are meant for joy and happiness in this life. Believe it and enjoy each and every day.

Kelly Lowe

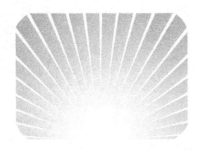

Special Additions

Jeff Primack's
RED PEPPER PASTE RECIPE

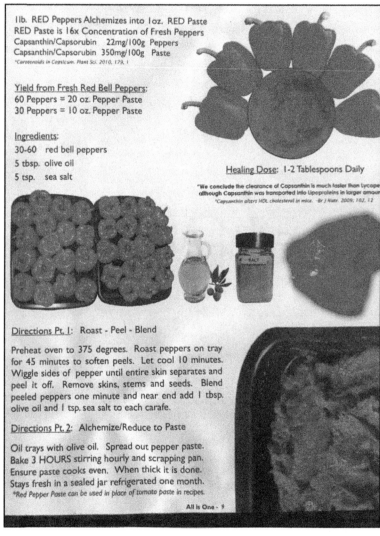

1lb. RED Peppers Alchemizes into 1oz. RED Paste
RED Paste is 16x Concentration of Fresh Peppers
Capsanthin/Capsorubin   22mg/100g Peppers
Capsanthin/Capsorubin 350mg/100g Paste
*Carotenoids in Capsicum. Plant Sci. 2010, 179, 1

Yield from Fresh Red Bell Peppers:
60 Peppers = 20 oz. Pepper Paste
30 Peppers = 10 oz. Pepper Paste

Ingredients:
30-60   red bell peppers
5 tbsp. olive oil
5 tsp.   sea salt

Healing Dose: 1-2 Tablespoons Daily

"We conclude the clearance of Capsanthin is much faster than Lycopene
although Capsanthin was transported into lipoproteins in larger amounts
*Capsanthin alters HDL cholesterol in mice. -Br J Nutr. 2009; 102, 12

Directions Pt. 1: Roast - Peel - Blend

Preheat oven to 375 degrees. Roast peppers on tray
for 45 minutes to soften peels. Let cool 10 minutes.
Wiggle sides of pepper until entire skin separates and
peel it off. Remove skins, stems and seeds. Blend
peeled peppers one minute and near end add 1 tbsp.
olive oil and 1 tsp. sea salt to each carafe.

Directions Pt. 2: Alchemize/Reduce to Paste

Oil trays with olive oil. Spread out pepper paste.
Bake 3 HOURS stirring hourly and scrapping pan.
Ensure paste cooks even. When thick it is done.
Stays fresh in a sealed jar refrigerated one month.
*Red Pepper Paste can be used in place of tomato paste in recipes.

All is One - 9

Used by permission, from
Food-Healing Cooking with Qi by Jeff Primack

Special Bonus:
Excerpted Chapters
From Kelly Lowe's First Book,

An Astrologer's Journey
My Life with the Stars

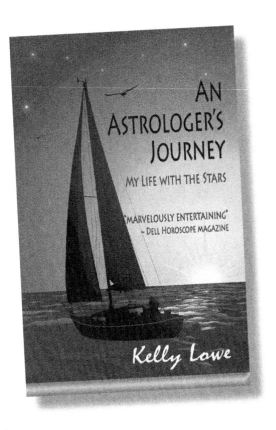

Kelly's first book, *An Astrologer's Journey, My Life With The Stars*, is an entertaining and inspiring ride through a life guided by the stars. You don't have to "speak astrology" to enjoy the journey. It is filled with real stories of how astrology helps so many to sail with favorable winds on life's changing seas. You can buy Kelly's books online at Amazon or Barnes and Noble, or on her website at www. astrologytalk.com.

*"All the world's a stage,
and all the men and women merely players;
they have their exits and their entrances,
and one man in his time plays many parts."*
~ Shakespeare, *As You Like It*

CHAPTER TWO

THE SEARCH FOR MYSELF

Drifting, drifting, drifting …

It was the early 1980s when I made a career move to Stuart, Florida. With no family, no friends, and no emotional support within two hundred miles, I felt like a ship adrift without an anchor. I was totally alone without friends or family close by.

I was looking forward to my new adventure in sales and marketing at this luxurious waterfront resort. It even had a marina where I could dock my sail boat. I was looking forward to my new position, which involved developing a sales and marketing plan to bring group and convention business to the resort.

Although I loved my job, which required long hours,

I continued to feel very alone and isolated when the day came to an end. I guess that is what motivated me to seek outside interests other than work and sailing.

I was fortunate. The local college offered a variety of different and unusual subjects, one of which was astrology. This was long before astrology was as mainstream as it is today. Since I was single and looking for "Mr. Right," I had picked up a couple of "astrological compatibility" books at the bookstores over the years. When I saw the opportunity to actually take a class and learn more about astrology, I was really excited.

I also took classes in Spanish, real-estate and how to fly an airplane—although I must admit that the astrology class was the only one that stuck with me. I never learned to speak Spanish, and I never learned how to fly an airplane. Nor did I pursue a career in real-estate.

What I did learn was fascinating and satisfying, and seemed to answer a lot of questions I had about things I was experiencing in my life. Although I didn't master the Spanish language, I did learn another language, the "Language of Astrology." And what a captivating language it turned out to be. Little did I realize it at the time, but astrology would soon open a whole new world for me—a world in which understanding myself, my family, my co-workers and friends wasn't such a mystery. What I learned, to my initial amazement, was that results here in this world are a direct product of when something is initiated. Timing, it turns out, really is everything.

It would be a mistake to imagine me in those days as some kind of "spiritual seeker" searching for a connection with the universe, or seeking the meaning of life. The truth is that I was just trying to get to know myself better and figure out why I do the things I do, and why I was feeling so unsure about everything. I didn't want lofty wisdom about the supernatural, eternity, or the spiritual realm. Later on in life I would ask such questions of myself, but at this point I wanted something concrete, and astrology offered concrete explanations.

As a result of this class and my own studies I was eager to seek a professional interpretation of my astrology chart. I inquired about making an appointment for an astrological consultation with my teacher at the college, but she was not seeing new clients at that time. However, she did refer me to a woman who lived in Hollywood, Florida. When I called Brenda to make my first astrology consultation appointment, she asked for my date, time and place of birth.

"SINCE THEN, THE CLOSER I HAVE LOOKED, THE MORE ASTROLOGY HAS MADE SENSE— NOT JUST IN GENERAL, BUT IN ALMOST EVERY INSTANCE IT HAS TESTED POSITIVE ..."

The hour-and-a-half drive from Stuart to Hollywood was filled with anticipation and excitement. What was this stranger going to tell me? Would she be able to help me sort out the dilemmas that I was experiencing in my life? Was she going to recognize that my life was in turmoil? Was she going to see that I was in my season of discontent? Would she see that I wanted to sell everything I owned and take off to sail around the world on my sailboat? That, although I had relocated and made a career change, I was still like a ship without an anchor? I was adrift. I felt that something was about to happen or that a change was coming in my life but I didn't know what, or when it was going to happen.

I was going to see Brenda with so many questions in my mind. I was seeking direction and answers. I wanted to better understand myself and why I was feeling the restlessness that troubled me so. But I was also feeling hopeful. Because the usual answers from the mainstream had failed to give me peace, and because I had already started studying astrology at the college, I went to see Brenda without a bit of skepticism. I was ready to listen, learn, and apply her insightful information. I was eager to learn.

Since then, the closer I have looked, the more astrology has made sense—not just in general, but in almost every instance it has tested positive when I compared what it indicated might happen and what actually did happen in my life and the lives of my friends, family and clients. Since that day in Brenda's office, I have understood and appreciated myself much more. Of course, I've faced life's usual problems, but I never again felt I had nowhere to turn for answers or explanations.

I still remember as if it were yesterday the moment that I walked into her office. Although I had given her only my birth information—date, time and place—over the phone when I made the appointment, it appeared that she already knew me very well.

Prior to my arrival she had calculated my astrological chart by placing all of the planets in the respective signs and degrees where they had been positioned at the time and place of my birth. She then placed the planets in the respective houses. Of course I didn't realize exactly what all of this meant at the time since I had not yet learned all the nuances of this new language.

From this chart Brenda was able to describe my personality, my likes and dislikes, and my family background. From my astrology chart, which she had prepared before I arrived, she could see that I was the first born in my family and that I had taken on responsibility at an early age. She could see that I was a very responsible person and that I took myself very seriously. She could see that my father had been in the military and I had traveled extensively to foreign countries in my youth. She could see that my love of travel carried over into my adult life, which led me to become a flight attendant and later seek a career in the hotel business which afforded me opportunity to continue my love for traveling the world.

She explained upfront that this astrological consultation was going to be about my past, present and future. I immediately thought, "How exciting is that?" This is going to be all about *me*. She explained that the past is important because astrology is about the study of cycles, and cycles repeat themselves. So by going back to the last time a cycle took place and remembering how we reacted to it or used it, we can benefit from the cycle when it repeats itself.

She then explained that I was currently experiencing one of the most critical and important cycles in my life. As you can imagine, that really got my attention! I knew that there was something really big going on in my life, but I just couldn't put my finger on what it was. Maybe this would explain the discontent and restlessness that I was feeling.

She explained that Saturn, the planet that rules structure, discipline and responsibility was traveling through my 4th house of home and family matters. This meant that I needed to get in touch with my roots, with my innermost personal life. It was an excellent time for psychotherapy or other consciousness raising, consciousness expanding studies. She said it might also bring about a change in residence.

Since the 4th house is the parental axis in the chart, this is also the time when you may have to take on a parental responsibility for someone, or take care of one of your parents. She explained that this would be a tremendous growth cycle for me. A "growth cycle" sounded exciting, but I later learned what that really meant. It meant suck it up and do whatever you need to do, because for the next couple of years life was not going to be a bowl of cherries.

That was news to me. I had been thinking that my next move might be to quit my job and sail around the world on my boat. It was during this time in my life that I read the classic book, *Sailing Alone around the World*. This was a sailing memoir by Joshua Slocum about his single-handed global circumnavigation in 1899. As it turned out, that adventure was not to be in my future.

As for my future? Brenda told me that I had Uranus in my 11th house. Of course I had no conception of what that meant, so she translated into simple English. She explained that it was one of the signatures in a chart of an astrologer. She said that I could easily go on to study and work in the field of astrology. This was an area of talent and strength for me. Now that was exciting information! My hopes resonated with that thought. I *did* feel that I was somehow connected to this cosmic science. The very idea of studying and learning more about this new language was exhilarating. Since I had majored in psychology in college, I was very interested in learning another tool with which to analyze myself and others.

I had come in to see Brenda with a lot of ideas in my head about who I was and where I was headed, but none of them felt like the true *me*, none of them fully satisfied me. Now I felt closer to having a true direction. I could feel a new kind of warmth inside, but at the same time I remembered Brenda's words. What would "a growth cycle" turn out to mean?

Kelly Lowe

"Be at peace and see a clear pattern and plan
running through all your lives.
Nothing is by chance."
~ Eileen Caddy, ***Footprints on the Path***

CHAPTER THREE

THE ADVENTURE BEGINS

Running with the Wind

My father was still a fairly young man and had always appeared to be in good health. In fact he was still working and leading an active and busy life. So you can imagine my shock and dismay when I received an emergency phone call from my mother while I was on a sales trip to Denver, Colorado. My father had suffered a heart attack. At that moment if someone had asked me for my name, I couldn't have answered them, but I did remember very clearly what Brenda had told me during our appointment: "I was about to take on a parental role."

My life was certainly going to change, that much I understood, but to what extent I still could not imagine. What would happen to my aspirations of quitting my job and sailing around the world? I didn't really have time to stop and mourn the end of that dream. My father's life and well-being instantly became my main priorities. Fortunately, the heart attack was not fatal, but he was going to require a great deal of home care before he would be strong enough to endure a heart bypass.

Since my mother was still working and I had been feeling very dissatisfied with my current life, it seemed only logical that I would be the family member to move back home and take care of my father. There was something about this scenario that really appealed to me. I knew in my heart that I was doing what I needed and wanted to do. The consultation with Brenda had given me the insight into my personality and the understanding of the cycle of life that I was in, so that I could happily embrace the task at hand and the opportunity to spend that quality time with my father.

"WITH ASTROLOGY I COULD SEE HOW SPECIFIC CONNECTIONS ACROSS TIME AND SPACE AFFECT EVENTS IN DAILY LIFE."

After my life-changing appointment with Brenda in Hollywood, I really became enthralled with this new language and new world that I had discovered. I knew there was truly some connection to the planets for us living on the earth. I could feel cosmic connection in my bones. To say my interest had been sparked would be a complete understatement. In that moment I realized that although my eyesight was 20/20, I had been blindly sleep-walking through life. Now I was beginning to wake up—and to look up. The word "Buddha" means one who is fully awake, and Jesus said spiritual connection requires a mystic rebirth "from above." I never once thought of myself as a prophet or teacher like the Buddha or Jesus, but in that moment I understood that there are infinite possibilities to life that I was just beginning to comprehend. I felt compelled to learn more about this mysterious, intriguing cosmic science called astrology.

So, even after moving away from Stuart, Florida, where I had completed my introduction to astrology class, I continued to expand my studies and seek knowledge whenever and wherever I could.

It was during this cycle in my life, that I took a Transcendental Meditation (TM) class and began the practice of daily meditation. I was introduced to the work of Edgar Cayce, one of the most prolific psychics in the twentieth century. I studied Tarot Cards, dream analysis, and numerology in addition to continuing my astrology studies.

And then came an exciting breakthrough. I met a woman named Betty Riley who helped change my life. She was a psychic medium who had written a book called *A Veil Too Thin—Out of Control*. Her true experience of reincarnation is one of the best documented cases on record. Without going too deeply into Betty Riley's story, she was a psychic of remarkable ability whose awareness of her past lives manifested in her present life. Her ability to see things far beyond the limitations of most people was so powerfully real that university researchers sought to find a viable explanation. So, when Betty saw something in me that I had not seen in myself, and encouraged me to pursue my astrological gifts, I knew that my path had been chosen. And, as I envisioned taking my life's work to a higher level, I also understood that the thing which made it a *higher* level was the opportunity for helping and working with others.

It was through my metaphysical studies, Betty's encouragement, and the seed that Brenda had planted during that first appointment that my interest and passion for astrology grew. After years of studying and observing the movement of the planets as they affect me and the lives of my family and friends, my avocation eventually was to become my vocation. My focus had moved beyond the search for myself; I had been given a gift and I knew it was meant to be shared.

As an astrology counselor, I feel that I am standing on solid ground. People throughout history have looked to the "heavens" as a way of explaining why things happen as they do, but so often the best they can come up with is, "It must have been God's will." Those can be comforting words but they don't really say much, and are usually uttered after the fact. That has never been enough for me. With astrology I could see how specific connections across time and space affect events in daily life—in the past, present, and future.

So I began my journey in earnest. I bought what seemed like a truckload of astrology books and continued with my studies. This was before the internet. I attended astrology conferences and conventions whenever I could. I studied with a mentor for several years and took a series of classes whenever and wherever I could.

"Be realistic: Plan for a miracle."
~ Bhagwan Shree Rajneesh

CHAPTER SEVEN

EXPANSION, OPTIMISM AND DISCIPLINE

From Jupiter to Saturn

Experiencing life is like riding a wave on the ocean. It's like watching the Sun rise and set. You might be busy preparing for a storm or enjoying a warm sunny day on the beach. Or it can be like preparing for a sunny day and getting a storm instead. Despite all of the elements which seem repetitious or familiar, life is constantly presenting us with something new. We are constantly building, preparing and repairing our lives. With the help of astrology we can do it better. It can be less painful, more gratifying and more predictable. Life truly is a journey, and through the use of astrology you can enjoy the ride more comfortably.

There will always be ups and downs, bumps in the road, good days and bad days, but understanding and working with your astrology chart can certainly prepare you for all of life's trials and tribulations.

Astrology can help you take advantage of the positive, advantageous good cycles that are coming up and it can help you prepare for and work through the difficult, more challenging cycles.

You could say that life accumulates as we live through these cycles. Hopefully we learn from them and discover how to take better advantage of the best and worst of times. It has been my desire for many years to compile my personal and professional experiences—the lessons learned through trials and tribulations which have guided me and my clients through this journey called life. In one sense, astrology is an experience of seeing ourselves in a larger context, of stepping far enough back from all the details which tend to cloud the big picture. Remembering that our natal chart is a picture of the sky at our moment of birth, there's great comfort in knowing there is an order to the universe that can be identified and understood, and that life is not just a series of random and disconnected moments. If we don't fight against these influences, if we let the universe have its way, things will generally turn out as they should and we will live a more fulfilled and stress free life.

Since this is a journey through my experiences, and since it always feels better to begin with the positive and pleasant experiences, that is exactly what I am going to do.

I can recall many years ago thinking about wanting to write a book. So I enrolled in a creative writing class at Rollins College. It was my heart's desire to share my experiences as they related to life's journey and the connection there is with astrology. But I guess I had not acquired enough of life's experience, nor was I ready to undertake what seemed to be too daunting a task. But now the saying "all things in their own time" has been proven valid once again, and my time for laying out the wisdom of my lessons learned is finally imminent.

THE JUPITER CONNECTION

One of the most enjoyable cycles that a person can experience is the cycle of Jupiter connecting with their Sun. This takes place approximately every 12 years. Unless there is some other overwhelmingly difficult cycle that is taking place at the same time, this can be one of the best times in a person's life.

After many years of being single and kissing a lot of frogs, I finally met my *Prince Charming* when transiting Jupiter was approaching my natal Sun. Since I was a student of astrology at the time, I appreciated the timing and significance of this relationship.

I had learned from my astrology studies—and experienced in my personal life—that this was considered one of the most benefic and enjoyable transits. To clarify in English, the word transit simple refers to the movement of a traveling planet across the sky. I knew that this was to be the beginning of a marvelous cycle. It was a wonderful time to initiate something new and expand my horizons. And it was a great time to broaden my perspective.

And that is exactly what I did. When transiting Jupiter was exactly at the same degree as my natal Sun, Larry and I were married.

In 2005 when Jupiter was traveling though my 3rd house of communications and writing I was inspired and motivated (the influence of Jupiter) to begin writing a book. Although the timing was right astrologically and my intentions and desire were there at the time, other priorities took precedence and the book was put on the back burner. Perhaps I had still not acquired enough experience and discipline to continue the task at that time.

At the writing of this book, Jupiter was traveling through my 9th house which rules teaching, publication and inspiration. I was definitely motivated and inspired. My motivation and inspiration were reinforced by the fact that my natal Sun in my 9th house was being transited by Jupiter. In simple English this means that Jupiter was traveling at the same degree as my natal Sun. This added a strong support to the mission at hand.

Although I would not say that astrology *predicts* the future, it can predict a favorable—or unfavorable—climate for the timing of success. Life is so much better when we can plan to do things at the most beneficial time, which correlates to the astrological cycles in our lives. Since I have always been a swimmer, I like to compare this to swimming downstream rather then swimming upstream. Sailing is another good analogy of the benefits of astrology. A responsible sailor wouldn't think of setting sail without checking the weather first. I can recall only too well the importance of checking the tide tables before trying to sail or motor sail under a bridge. Several years ago, while living in South Florida, I almost ran my sailboat into a bridge as I was trying to motor sail under the bridge against the tide. It's always good to know which way the tide is flowing when you are making your plans in life.

JUPITER AND INSPIRATIONAL CONNECTIONS — YOUR GUARDIAN ANGELS

Strike while the iron is hot. Jupiter, the planet of abundance can be inspiring and motivating … and if someone comes along with their Sun in the same sign as your Jupiter, it can be magical for you both. You don't know why; you just connect with each other. Often times this person will play an inspirational or motivational role in your life, and you will do the same in theirs as well. These are people who will often promote you, or help you accomplish your dreams and goals. We can't really seek them out, or run an ad on the internet for them. They just seem to come into your life exactly when you need them. They recharge your battery, uplift your spirits and motivate you. I like to call them guardian angels.

"LIFE IS SO MUCH BETTER WHEN WE CAN PLAN TO DO THINGS AT THE MOST BENEFICIAL TIME, WHICH CORRELATES TO THE ASTROLOGICAL CYCLES IN OUR LIVES."

I am blessed with many guardian angles in my life, some of whom I have become more aware of than others. As an astrologer, I am more inclined than most people to ask a new acquaintance for their birth date when I start associating with them—especially if we are going to develop any kind of a business relationship. But sometimes these angels just show up unanticipated in a social setting and before you know it they have become instrumental in inspiring and promoting you. When you find out later that you have a strong connection, such as a Jupiter/Sun connection, it really doesn't come as a surprise.

Guardian angels can arrive when you least expect them. Joann came to me out of the blue at a golf event. We were attending a social networking breakfast with the Executive Women's Golf Association, where she had a display table for her cosmetic business. I happened to be interested in her product and she was interested in astrology. As our friendship developed she invited me to join NCW, a professional women's networking group that she was a member of. Since I was new to the area and had not met many people, I really did not have a good connection to the business community. So, excited to meet new people and expand my horizons, I joined Networking Connects Women, without any expectations as to where it would take me.

As luck would have it, this group of women turned out to be a wonderful source of networking—much more so than I could ever have hoped for. It was comfortable and easy to develop personal and business relationships with the women. There were many professional services and businesses represented among them, from a wonderful jeweler to an excellent massage therapist whose services I was delighted to avail myself of.

One of the members, Christine, who was the publisher of a local magazine, suggested that I start doing monthly astrology lectures at a local restaurant. She had a contact at a restaurant in town that was interested in sponsoring the event. We decided to call it "Dinner with the Stars."

This was the first time I had done anything publicly since moving to my new home town. As it turned out, this became a springboard which opened a whole new avenue for me. I had the opportunity to introduce astrology to people I otherwise might never have met. My Jupiter/Sun connection with my guardian angel Joann continues to be an inspirational connection and friendship.

Another guardian angel, Krista, was a member of the professional women's networking group. She owns and operates the Daytona Yoga & Wellness Center. Since I have always been drawn to yoga, I was immediately attracted to her. We quickly became friends and kindred spirits. When she invited me to do astrology workshops at her studio, I was delighted. Here again, this opportunity opened the way for me to meet many like-minded, beautiful souls. My Jupiter/Sun connection with Krista also continues to be an inspirational connection and friendship.

One day, while I was in the midst of getting started with writing this book, I was surprised by an unsolicited email from guardian angel Krista. She forwarded me a notice she had received about a workshop titled, "Independent Book Publishing—Six Steps to Success." I immediately rearranged my schedule so that I could attend the workshop, which happened to be taking place the very next day. The timing was perfect. It was exactly what I was looking for and I was not disappointed.

When I arrived at the studio on the day of the workshop, I immediately noticed a tall, striking gentleman standing toward the front of the room with whom I felt an instant connection. I was not surprised to learn that he was conducting the workshop. As the class began I couldn't help wondering what his Sun sign might be, or what connection we might have in our astrological charts. So at the conclusion of the workshop I asked him about his birthday. Since I had identified myself as an astrologer during the introductions, I felt that it gave me the liberty to be so bold to ask him. He didn't seem to object, although he did whisper the year in my ear. I immediately recognized that his Sun sign was conjunct by Jupiter which I shared with him.

His puzzled and bewildered look again reminded me that astrology is a language onto itself and most people do not speak it. So, using simple non-astrological English, I quickly tried to explain that we shared an astrological connection, in that his Sun sign was in the same sign as my Jupiter. This was a very interesting and positive connection. Since I was on a time crunch to leave and there were other people from the class waiting to speak with him, I tried to make the explanation as concise as possible. I took his card and casually said I would look at his chart as I was interested in how we might hit it off working together. I would get back with him to perhaps ask him to help me with my book. But at that point I already knew that I had met another guardian angel. I knew that he was going be instrumental in editing and helping me publish my book.

Guarding angels do seem to arrive when you least expect them and exactly when you need them most. It has happened to me so often that I really have started expecting them to be there for me. Wouldn't it be interesting if everyone had their astrological Sun sign and the sign their Jupiter was in at the time they were born displayed on their forehead? This would enable everyone to instantly identify their guardian angels and they could identify you. However, I do believe that we are intuitively attracted to those people who are inspirational and helpful to us. They often remain in our lives indefinitely.

GIRLFRIENDS FOREVER

Some people pass through your life like a ship in the night, while others remain as pillars of stability and friendship that can last a life time.

Such was the case of two dynamic, special women who have been supportive and lasting friends in my life for many years. I have always believed that there are no such thing as coincidence. I believe that we meet everyone at the right time, in the right place and just when we are supposed to meet them.

When Jupiter, the planet of optimism and expansion, was traveling through my 11th house I decided to join our local Toastmasters organization. The 11th house deals with groups, clubs and organizations, and with getting in touch with your hopes, goals, dreams and wishes. I had always wanted to be a public speaker. Since I knew that timing was everything, I chose this particular cycle to develop my speaking skills and my confidence. I wanted to become more socially interactive and share my experiences with astrology in a more public forum. It was my intention to eventually speak about astrology in a light and entertaining way at conventions and organizations. I knew this would be an excellent time to take on this study.

As it turned out, it wasn't very long before I was speaking at conventions, clubs, groups and organizations throughout the state.

Once you begin experiencing how the movement of the planets influences us, you no longer hope for the desired outcome, you simply expect it and gain confidence in what you are doing. So I sailed on, feeling assurance that this would be a productive time for me to take the understanding of life I had gained from astrology out into the larger world.

As I worked through the Toastmasters manual, diligently learning how to prepare my speeches, I was befriended by Liz, who was to become my mentor. It just so happened that Liz and I had a Sun/Jupiter connection. Her Sun was at the same degree and sign as my Jupiter. As I mentioned before, this usually proves to be a very uncomplicated, enjoyable, beneficial and long lasting friendship.

As luck or "the stars" would have it, Liz not only mentored me though my Toastmasters speeches, she also introduced me to an entirely new circle of woman friends. She was a member of Beta Sigma Phi, a women's professional sorority which happened to be pledging new members.

This is where I met Rita, a long-time dear friend of Liz's. Notice I don't say "old friend." She would never forgive me. I wasn't surprised to learn that Rita's Moon was in the same degree and sign as my Jupiter. This is also an indication of an endearing, long-lasting friendship. So Liz, Rita and I enjoyed the bond of a strong Jupiter/Sun/Moon connection. It is no surprise that the three of us have remained close friends for more than twenty-five years.

Of course, I didn't know it or even think about it at the time, but forming lifelong friendships and a mutual support network with this special group of women in the professional sorority was the epitome of "swimming downstream." It all came together naturally, as if it was meant to be. Which it was! When my husband, Larry was diagnosed with congestive heart failure and suffered a fatal heart attack, they were by my side every step of the way. They arrived in full force at his memorial service and continued to hold my hand as I recovered from my loss.

Life offers many gifts as we make our journey. But one of the greatest gifts is the people we meet who have a connection with our Jupiter.

LOVE STORY

He was going to be an actor; she was going to save the world. There was an instant chemistry and attraction. Even though they were young, barely sixteen, they knew they had something special between them. What they didn't know was what life paths were in store for them.

They grew up in a small town in the Midwest. Both went their separate ways after high school. They promised to keep in touch. This was before cell phones, texting and internet were the rage. They continued to meet at holidays and summer vacations, but it soon became apparent that their lives were going in different directions. But even so, they felt this deep-seated bond between them.

You see, her Venus was in the same degree and Sun sign as his Jupiter. This is a very favorable connection between two people. It promotes a peaceful and harmonious relationship. It reduces the couple's feeling of stress and encourages a desire for peace and forgiveness. This is one of the most enduring and loving connections two people can have. The other is when two people have a Sun/Venus connection in their charts.

So not only did they feel very comfortable when they were together, but they could never be mad at each other. But as time passed on, their chosen career paths led them in different directions. He was living in New York and she in Colorado. Eventually she met someone else. They lost contact when she became engaged.

Shortly after she said "I do," she began to feel that something was missing in her marriage, but she could never quite put her finger on it. After 14 years, when Saturn made its difficult aspect in her marriage chart, the marriage could not withstand the pressure. They separated and eventually divorced.

After the dust had settled and she recovered from the emotional trauma of the divorce, she started thinking about her old friend and adolescent sweetheart. Or maybe she never stopped thinking about him. This was also about the time that she was preparing to attend her class reunion. Yes, her special friend with whom she had such a strong Jupiter/Venus connection also attended the reunion.

It was as though no time had passed since they last saw each other. He had never married and she was once again single. They instantly reconnected. Although they still lived miles apart, cell phones and the internet made the distance seem insignificant. Their endearing, enduring friendship and budding romance were once again on track.

SATURN AND THE MARRIAGE CYCLE

They had what appeared to be a perfect marriage. Both were well educated. She was a Libra Sun and he a Gemini Sun. Their strong emphasis of the air signs in their charts indicated their tendency to have the characteristic of being mentally acute, active, social and outgoing. Their lives seemed to be right on track, both with promising careers, an active social life and a beautiful home and family. Gemini, Libra, and Aquarius are known as the air signs. (*see Words to Guide You … Page XII*)

They were certainly mentally and intellectually compatible and they parented a very intelligent child. In the beginning they enjoyed the outdoors: hiking, skiing, sailing, jogging. But as with many happy couples, they began to drift apart. The first signs of discontent starting surfacing around the seven-year mark of their marriage. As it turned out, that was also the time that Saturn presented its first difficult aspect in their wedding chart. That difficult aspect is what is called a "Saturn square."

It is not unusual for a marriage to experience challenges at this time. Couples often have to work through issues that have been building over the past seven years. It may present itself as a financial challenge, or as a cycle of discontent. It's a time when a relationship can either become stronger or dissolve. My professional experience over the years has taught me that this is often when someone will seek counseling—or an attorney.

Albert and Wanda survived the first difficult patch,

"the seven year itch," but the next hard Saturn cycle which came seven years later was not going to be so easy. They had both developed very busy lives which seemed to pull them in different directions. Neither of them had found another love interest; they had just drifted apart and became physically incompatible. They knew that their marriage was not working any more.

Interestingly, statistics show that the seven- and fourteen-year marks in a marriage are the most critical. Although they were still friends, they knew they didn't want to be married to each other any longer.

Saturn, the tester and teacher in the chart, tested them to the limit. Fortunately, they were able to draw on their strong Libra and Gemini Suns—Libra being the peacemaker and Gemini the information processor—and were able to maintain a friendship and arbitrate a "friendly divorce." Working through a mediator with no attorneys, they came to an amenable agreement and moved on with their lives. A Saturn cycle doesn't last forever, so take comfort in remembering that we always learn from them and the Saturn cycles help us appreciate the easier, usually more pleasant, Jupiter cycles.

We always seem to remember so vividly the challenging times in our lives, but let's remember to appreciate and enjoy the good times.

THE LANGUAGE OF ASTROLOGY, ABRIDGED

Words to Guide You on Kelly's Journey

(If you are unfamiliar with the language of astrology,
you may find this brief "glossary" helpful.)

Your Chart – Everyone has one. Your astrology chart is the picture of the sky at the moment and place you were born. It speaks volumes about who you are. If you don't like your chart and always wished you were born under a different sign, blame your parents—or the stars—not your Astrology Counselor.

Natal Planet – Where a planet was at the time of your birth, not the planet on which you were born. Most of us were born on earth, and those who weren't usually won't admit it.

Let Your Sun Sign In – Your Sun sign refers to the sign of the zodiac that your Sun was in at the moment and time of your birth. Your Sun sign describes your personality. If you don't like your personality, you can't hire a lawyer and change your Sun sign like changing your name. My advice is don't fight it, use it. There are wonderful possibilities in all the signs.

Aries – pioneering, independent, competitive, intolerant, aggressive

Taurus – patient, steadfast, conservative, materialistic, thorough

Gemini – literary, versatile, adaptable, analytical, curious

Cancer – self-sacrificing, receptive, cautious, reserved, persevering

Leo – commanding, generous, ambitious, optimistic, opinionated

Virgo – ingenious, witty, studious, methodical, skeptical

Libra – persuasive, tactful, intriguing, undecided, judicial

Scorpio – secretive, penetrating, intellectual, investigative, temperamental

Sagittarius – jovial, progressive, philosophical, frank, zealous

Capricorn – laborious, forceful, scrupulous, thrifty, domineering

Aquarius – inventive, intellectual, diplomatic, independent, humanitarian

Pisces – intuitive, compassionate, introspective, loquacious, clairvoyant

My House or Yours – Understanding the houses in your chart takes you deeper into the language of astrology. Have you heard it said that accidents often happen in your own house? Well, good things happen there too. Knowing your chart can help determine how your story plays out.

In Western Astrology the astrological chart is divided into 12 houses. A house is an arc in space that represents 30 degrees. Hence, 12 houses equals 360 degrees. Each house represents an area of your life. And each house has a ruling planet, which is also known as a correlating planet ruler. I know that's a lot to grasp, but remember this: The houses tell us **"where"** something is going to happen.

1st house: Aries, Mars—your physical body

2nd house : Taurus, Venus —your finances and values

3rd house: Gemini, Mercury—your education and the way you communicate

4th house : Cancer, Moon—your home and family

5th house: Leo, Sun—your children, your love life, and your creativity.

6th house: Virgo, Mercury—your health and your work environment

7th house: Libra, Venus—your marriage or partnerships

8th house: Scorpio, Pluto—your sex life, inherence and joint finances

9th house: Sagittarius, Jupiter—your higher education and philosophy

10th house: Capricorn, Saturn—your career and public image

11th house: Aquarius, Uranus—your hopes, goals, dreams and wishes

12th house: Pisces, Neptune—your subconscious attitudes

Ascendant – Your ascendant is the Sun sign that was on the horizon at the moment and place that you were born. It is referred to as your "window to the world." If your Sun sign doesn't seem to completely describe you, peeking out "your window" might help you see your world more clearly. Don't be afraid to look. What you see might be a pleasant surprise.

Transits – Planets are always on the move. Transits are the constant rotation of the planets as they orbit the Sun. As they enter a house they tell us **"when"** something is going to happen. This is especially obvious when following the transit of the Moon. If you unexpectedly find yourself falling in love, and you're not dancing the *bossa nova* or drinking margaritas, it may be the Moon to blame.

Aspect – refers to the relationship or distance of one planet from another. The aspect of planets acting together can alter or increase their individual influence. We begin to see there's more to the language of astrology than just knowing the difference between an earth sign and a water sign. Astrology counselors train many years—and sometimes shed many tears—before beginning their practice. So ... if you are an amateur sitting at home trying to render your boyfriend's chart ... well, let me just say we don't want anyone getting hurt. And finally ...

Planets in Action — In the language of astrology the Sun and Moon are both planets, no matter what your 8th grade science teacher might say.

Sun – your inner being

Moon – your emotions

Mercury – you mental perception

Venus – your attitude about love and your self worth

Mars – your energy level

Jupiter – your guardian angel

Saturn – your tester and teacher

Pluto – your transformer

Uranus – your intuition

Neptune – your compassion

Elements — Each Sun sign is assigned an element which helps describe its characteristics. The elements are Fire, Earth, Air and Water

AIRES, LEO AND SAGITTARIUS are the *Fire* signs—known for their feisty high spirited energy.

GEMINI, LIBRA AND AQUARIUS are the *Air* signs—known for their mental and intellectual equity.

TAURUS, VIRGO, AND CAPRICORN are the *Earth* signs—known for their logical, concrete and practical nature.

CANCER, SCORPIO AND PISCES are the *Water* signs—known for their sensitivity and keen intuition.

Kelly Lowe

CPSIA information can be obtained
at www.ICGtesting.com
Printed in the USA
LVOW03s0319220118
563397LV00001B/1/P